To: my b

From. Her

Je

Dr Harry Cooper graduated from Sydney University Veterinary School in 1965. Since that time he has practised in Australia and in Great Britain. Today he lives with his wife Janine and their daughter Heidi on sixty-five rolling acres at Relbia in the north of Tasmania. It is both a working farm and the set for much of 'Harry's Practice'. Many of the animals seen in the series live and breed on the farm. There are five stallions at stud, an Arabian, two Welsh Section As, a Riding Pony and a Paint. Seven or eight foals are born each year and there are many visiting mares as well. The cattery breeds show-quality Burmese, Siamese and Devon Rex and boards up to twenty-five cats in heated runs. Cavalier King Charles spaniels, Racing Greyhounds and Miniature fox terriers are regularly bred also. At the present time there are thirty-one horses and foals, twenty-nine cats and kittens, eighteen dogs and six pups, thirteen coloured sheep, twelve Muscovy ducks, seven Rex rabbits, three guinea pigs, almost thirty fantail pigeons, one cockatiel and around forty colourful goldfish. The workload is constant.

DR HARRY COOPER

Stethoscopes & Calving Ropes

DR HARRY COOPER

Stethoscopes & Calving Ropes

MACMILLAN
Pan Macmillan Australia

First published 2002 in Macmillan by Pan Macmillan Australia Pty Limited
St Martins Tower, 31 Market Street, Sydney

Reprinted 2002

National Library of Australia
cataloguing-in-publication data:

Cooper, Harry, 1944– .
Stethoscopes & calving ropes.
ISBN 0 7329 1153 2.

1. Cooper, Harry, 1944– – Anecdotes.
2. Veterinarians – Australia – Anecdotes. I. Title.

636.089092

My four-legged friends on the cover are: Rosalie the cow ('Merseybank Beretta Rosalie') courtesy of Geoff and Anne Hazelwood, Merseybank Jersey Stud, La Trobe, Tas; Otis the Red Burmese ('Creswell Inferno') courtesy of Janine and Harry Cooper, Relbia, Tas; Scarlett the Border Collie ('Wirrillawind La Petite'), courtesy of Wirrillawind Kennels, Mudgee, NSW.

Illustrations by Elliot Cowan

Typeset in Sabon 12/16 by Midland Typesetters
Printed in Australia by McPherson's Printing Group

To my parents to whom I owe so much,
To my family to whom I owe much more,
To our animals past and present,
to whom I owe my livelihood,
And to all the children of the world, may their love and
respect for their animals translate into a love and
understanding of their fellow man.

Contents

Introduction

This is the third and possibly the last book in what has been a re-living of the fifty-eight years of my life. Writing takes time. Good writing takes a lot longer. This last labour has been both a pleasure and an exercise in recollection that has strained every cell in that overtaxed brain within my balding skull.

I must thank my wife for her tolerance in the time taken to compile this book, and my stenographer Janice for her patient understanding of my Australianisms. Thanks also go to all the clients and friends within the animal-owning community, to my veterinary colleagues and to those persons still around who may have had their names and places changed to protect them from further embarrassment. Without all of you there would be no stories and there would be no book to write. Every tale is true. Each new day brings a different challenge and with it perhaps another chapter.

To my publishers, thanks for letting me get the manuscript in a little later than the deadline. The workload this year has been as heavy as always.

The locker has been emptied. It is time to take home what's left of the dirty washing and to leave the space as it once was. Neat and tidy. I've aired most of it, and trust that you have laughed a lot and cried a little, for that is what animals do to us all. If in reading this you have gained a greater knowledge of what has made Dr Harry and his family what they are today, then I am happy. I trust you like what you read – if not, be sure and tell me.

There will be other books in the future. Books for children and educative books as well. It is my prayer that mankind shall recognise that the Lord God gave us dominion over the animal kingdom. We must rule with patience, diligence, understanding and with perspective. The animals – whether you believe they were created or simply evolved – were here before us, and they deserve to remain. One day it will no longer be up to us. It will be up to our children. As Crosby, Stills, Nash and Young once sang, 'teach your children well'.

For the sake of our civilisation, please, do just that.

Dr Harry Cooper
Relbia, Tasmania

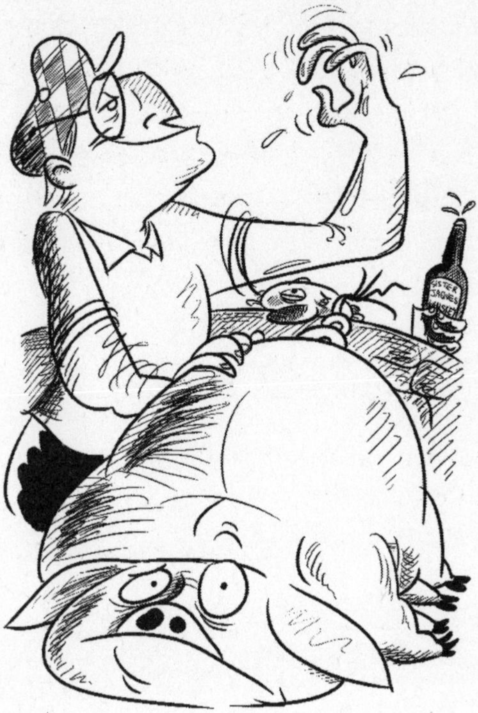

Looking Back

1

Mum and Dad

Without a doubt the biggest influence on my entire life has been my parents. Those of you who have read my previous volumes will no doubt be struck by the frequent references to them both. Even on 'Harry's Practice' I find myself constantly evoking their knowledge.

My mother was a lady of the theatre and had, over the years, bred Pomeranians. She was with the legendary J.C. Williamson Company for most of her life. Mum's pride and joy was a letter, handwritten in black ink on yellowing hand-crafted paper, carefully framed and hanging on the wall of their lounge room. It was from 'Our Glad' – Gladys Moncrieff – thanking her for the performances where Mum had stepped in as understudy in her leading role. From my mother came I believe the gift of performing, the love of standing in front of a live audience and telling a story. One such occasion was the garden show at Nambour.

Every year the promoters invited a special guest to speak. Not about gardening, heaven knows there were plenty of experts around to deal with that subject, but rather to break the mood and talk about something totally different. 'Talk to the Animals' was in full swing and it was my turn to have a go. The venue was an ageing grandstand, set on the edge of an oval. It had become the focus of the show and speakers took to the podium one after another. The event ran over three days.

I spoke once each day, usually around one o'clock. Seating was on hard wooden benches with very little in the way of back support, and it rose steeply from the narrow pathway that separated the front row from the almost antique scrolled ironwork of the facade. There were three aisles in all – the centre and at each end of the seat rows.

It was the last day. I was tired. Mixing with the public for three days straight is good fun but still hard work, and personal contact is very draining. The talk was all but over. In those days I concluded with my story about the gibbons I encountered in a zoo, and how a particular gibbon came to have such a meaningful conversation with me. (The story is in *Anecdotes & Antidotes*.) I was at the part where the gibbon comes down and puts his cheek next to mine, when suddenly, five rows back to the right of the centre aisle a listener burst into tears. The lady was totally oblivious to all around her, sitting there crying her eyes out. As an eerie hush descended over the entire audience, I stopped. She kept crying. Loudly now. Very loudly. Every person in that grandstand was looking at her.

Something inside me said, 'Do it'. I walked slowly up the aisle to where she was sitting, tapped her gently on the shoulder. She looked up, directly into my face. The floodgates opened again. I sat, right alongside her. She continued to sob. Deep chest-heaving sobs. I continued the story, telling it directly to her, pausing only when her crying became too loud to continue. My friends, this was not just the zoo keeper's gibbon, not just my gibbon, not your gibbon. It had become *her* gibbon – and the most magical moment in all my days of storytelling. Nobody moved; every person in that grandstand was focused on her. To hold an audience 'in the palm of your hand' is a most exhilarating feeling. Thanks, Mum.

From my father I learnt a love of all animals, an instinct to care and the ability to relate to people. This he taught me at an early age. The phone would ring and as children my brother and I were supposed to answer it correctly and hold a conversation with the usually unknown person on the other end until one parent or the other appeared. This was tough but good training.

Dad had wanted to be a vet. In his youth he had apprenticed himself to a practitioner, but had worked there only twelve months, for on taking his annual fortnightly vacation he was offered a job with a shipping company. He rose to be managing director and never went back to veterinary work.

He had contacts everywhere and could get anything for anyone. From him came my drive to become a vet. He only belted me twice. Once for throwing stones and the other for a poor school report – grade two at high school, Latin. I hated it. The report read '37% . . . failed . . . complacently careless'. Complacency was not in Dad's dictionary, and I hope and pray it's not in mine either. It was his unfulfilled desire to become a vet that drove his urge to see his two sons achieve what he had failed to do. 'I want to see you established,' he would say. Well, Dad, if they get Channel Seven up there I suppose you know what I'm up to, and, yes, I think my brother and I are both well established.

One funny thing I should report. Dad was a teetotaller. There was always beer in the fridge for the visitors but he never drank. My brother and I enjoyed both beer and wine once we were old enough, but always respected the family home and kept consumption down to a minimum. Dad died in his early eighties and he's been gone well over twenty years, so he'll not mind my sharing this story, I'm sure. It was time to clean up his personal possessions after the funeral. For my part, two pairs of gold cufflinks, ancient dog ribbons, some pictures taken throughout Dad's life, and the odd personal letter written during the wartime prior to my birth were souvenirs enough. There was plenty of him in me, anyway.

'What will we do with all this stuff?' my brother Neil asked, stacking yet another carton of Dad's favourite cough mixture on top of the other two.

'Throw it out, I reckon.' The stuff tasted dreadful, but Dad always had a bottle or two around for his constant catarrh. After buying it by the carton all that time, he'd even got to know the head chemist where they made it.

'Look at this label,' my brother said, reading out the list of contents. 'The preservative contains a fair percentage of alcohol.'

Bonnington's Irish Moss. 'The steady sip, sip, sip, of the pectoral oxymel of carrageen' went the commercial. Dad took the ad literally, and to his dying day I'm sure he never knew what was in the stuff. You do now, Dad!

2

Just Once Around

Some thirty years ago, when I was a relatively young vet working at Gladesville, there were two greyhound tracks operating in Sydney. Wentworth Park was as it still stands today, opposite the huge wool stores in Wattle Street and very close to the now-bustling fish markets. Sure, it has been updated somewhat since those days with several redesigns of the track and its surface, but it remains basically the same shape, a tight rapidly turning circle, with very short straights and sharp bends. A test of the dogs' ability to jump fast and rail. The shortest way home is along the rails and a dog needs to be smart on its feet to win here.

The other greyhound track was Harold Park, totally the opposite in design. Laid out inside the trotting track, it was a 'U-turn' pattern, with two very long parallel straights of over 200 metres each and a fairly tight bend at both ends. The dogs jumped right onto the straight, ran to the turn, and once around it, the post was another ten or eleven seconds away, if the race was 500 metres. Over the distance, 800 metres, it was one and a half times around. This was the speed track, a test of sheer pace and power.

It was a rare occurrence to see me at Harold Park, the dogs were so far away from the crowd, whereas at 'Wenty' you could almost reach out and touch them as they galloped past. But this night I'd been invited.

Sid didn't need to drive, he lived so close it took less than ten minutes to walk to the track. Kennelling time was fast approaching, but with his usual relaxed manner Sid and the dog were making their way slowly up the hill to the entry gate. A rather sad sight they made, an old man and his old dog, both walking with the shuffling gait that comes with the advancement of years. Sid with his head bowed from hours of toil in manual trades that today would be performed by machines in a matter of minutes. Billy, his faithful dog now reaching the twilight of his career as a four-year-old, seemed to find it an effort to climb the ramp up to the kennel area. I watched as they passed the familiar identification check and veterinary examination that all competitors had to undergo. Billy seemed almost asleep. Around him the younger dogs were barking and carrying on, infused with the energy of youth. He was an old hand. He knew that you save that energy for later, you may just need it.

Sid gathered up the simple blanket that would be Billy's bed in the kennel, as he waited for his race to be called. Soon they'd disappear into the kennel block proper. The old dog sniffed the familiar grey flannel as he'd done a hundred times before. Sid knelt for a minute, pulled the dog to him, a gentle pat on the head and a word in the dog's ear. Five minutes later he was back outside looking around at the gathering crowd.

'Sorry, mate, I didn't get a chance to say g'day before you kennelled him,' I apologised.

'Don't worry, son, he'll be fine, he'll be fine,' and off we went for a quiet beer before the night's racing began.

As a young vet it takes quite a time for established clients of the practice in which you are employed to 'trust' you with their animals. For some unknown reason, right from the first consultation there was none of that with Sid. 'You do the job right, son, and you'll do me.' To Sid I was always 'son', there was over forty years between us. He was a man of few words. With no more than one or two dogs in his kennel at a time, most of Sid's dogs became real pets. He would spend hours in their company just patting and talking to them. For many of the racing elite the old fella and his quaint ways were a bit of a joke.

When you work with animals, things soon start to become obvious – that is, as long as you take the time to observe them. These dogs of Sid's really appeared to listen to him. Their relationship, the dogs with the man and vice versa, was unique. Sid had the time and he made the time.

Billy had been a good dog, a really good dog. He had won well over thirty races in his career, the majority over the distance (meaning 600 to 800 metres). His talent had taken him to a track record in country New South Wales and several victories in invitation class races at Harold Park. Five months ago the black dog had suffered a severe muscle injury. The sort of thing that would end the career of lesser dogs.

There is a powerful muscle in both hind legs of the greyhound called the gracilis. It runs down the inside of the thigh from the groin to the back of the knee. It is one of the major propulsive elements of the hind leg. Damage to this area is called a 'dropped back muscle'. In racing the dog simply rips it in half, at the top or the bottom! Apart from broken bones, it is, I guess, the most significant injury a dog can sustain. Billy had almost totally torn off the top of this muscle.

'Whatever you reckon, son,' Sid glibly acknowledged with a nod of his head when I told him I wanted to try a repair.

'It'll be purely experimental, you know that,' I hastened to explain, 'but I can't see why we shouldn't have a try'. Endeavouring to justify a procedure often dreamed about but seldom undertaken. 'There's this new suture material I want to try, the stuff they use in heart transplants. It's like fishing line, a bit stretchy and the body doesn't react to it.' All of this technical rubbish was of no concern to Sid, or to Billy, who had his eye on the little poodle on the other side of the waiting room.

From a strictly surgical point of view the op went without a hitch.

'That's the easy bit, mate, the long slog is your department.' Sid was unfazed, as usual.

'This is a faradic stimulator, here's how it works,' I explained. Billy lay on the table as if asleep while I coupled up the electrodes. 'It will make the muscle twitch, and help to build up the bulk and avoid adhesions.' For a bloke with no technical training, Sid was no idiot. He only needed to be shown once!

Two months later, after several checks and loads of swimming and physiotherapy, it was time for Billy to go for a gallop. Watching from the centre of a football field, I felt this sensational buzz as Billy whirled and twirled on his bionic leg. The rehabilitation went well. In three months he was back racing. The first few starts were unremarkable, a place here and there but nothing near his old form, and then slowly the placings became a win or two, only over the 500 but he was pulling up sound. Tonight would really see what he was made of.

'We thought, the wife and I, that we'd nominate as a bit of a joke really,' Sid explained. 'I didn't expect to get a run.' I don't think anyone did. In fact, Billy (his racing name has long deserted my memory bank) was only drawn as a reserve. Not in his familiar distance, but in the top grade sprint of the night. He was there just to make up the field.

'Hell, mate, all those bloody speed machines, I don't know if the old fella is ready for it.'

Frankly, neither did I. Prolene is pretty good suture material, but would it take this sort of treatment?

'There were three scratchings all up, the six, the eight and the other reserve – blow me down, he's got the start from the eight!' Sid glanced at his fob watch, a farewell present from the foundry. Much battered, but an accurate timepiece.

'Better go, son, better go . . . Need to talk to Billy . . . Gotta go,' and he shuffled off in the direction of the kennels.

You could watch the dogs being inspected prior to racing in the rugging area; from there it's out to the parade ring for a quick toilet stop before the long walk to the starting boxes. Sid was slow and deliberate. The number nine, green and white striped rug of the first reserve slipped easily over the greying muzzle of the lanky black dog. It was knotted so carefully, and tied with a double bow as those gnarled hands smoothed the dog's silky hair and calmed his very being. Again he knelt by the dog and whispered into his ear, a hug around the neck and a stroke of the head. They were last into the parade area. Billy just sniffed the night air, the wooden post, cocked the damaged leg and turned back to Sid. All the others were leaping and prancing at the ends of their leads. Sid and Billy stood motionless. He leant down once again. They were close to me this time as I stood by the fence. The words were faint, but I'm sure I heard 'Just once around tonight, Billy, just once around tonight.' The old man's hand never stopped stroking his dog. Then they moved out onto the track for that most important walk of all. Last in line, Sid and Billy followed the field to the starting boxes.

The big black dog had won many a distance race here in his time, but tonight it would be different. This time he didn't have the extra 300 metres to unwind his punishing finish. This time it would be just once around. A mad dash on a leg of nylon, muscle and bone, against dogs far younger and brasher than he. My mouth was dry, it was an effort to swallow a huge lump that seemed to be welling up and choking the entrance of my larynx. Billy was special, he carried a bit of me in every nylon suture. If the old fella pulled up sound I'd be happy.

They reached the starting boxes at last. All the young things barked and twirled, all except Billy. He stood beside the man who loved him. A man and an animal, against a field that in his younger days he may very well have given a hammering. A man and a dog, as it has been for so many thousands of years. A man and a dog silhouetted against the night sky by the blaze of neon behind them. The rest of the field were walking back to the start. Sid knelt once again, and spoke with Billy. Perhaps he and I were the only people on the track that night to know what this message was to mean. The lids slammed shut on the boxes.

'One, three, five, seven,' called the starter, and the four dogs moved forward. 'Put 'em in,' and the dogs were carefully placed in and the doors locked behind. 'OK, two, four, eight.' Billy was right on the outside of the field, but also out of trouble. In an instant the old dog lit up. His ears pricked at, 'put 'em in', he didn't need to be told. Like the trouper he was, Billy went straight to the front of the boxes and assumed the familiar crouch that all good dogs have. As the lids open they can spring into stride.

The green light shone, the commentator broke into voice, the lure rolled and the three of us waited. Greyhound racing is so quick. They cover 300 metres in sixteen seconds. Twice the speed of a world-class human sprinter. The field began almost as one. The number one dog soon speared to the front with the two and three hot on his heels. The seven dog crossed quickly to the rails as there was no six dog and proceeded to flatten both the four and the five, on the inside of him, as he did. This left Billy with an uninterrupted run right down the outside of the first straight. It's well and good to be able to go flat out in a straight line but at Harold Park you have to get around one corner and it's a totally banked U-turn. Experienced dogs know how to handle it, the drag lure speed machines just can't manage it.

By the time the one dog was entering the turn, Billy was some eight or nine lengths behind in about fourth or fifth spot, and fairly wide on the track. The seven dog, having done a demolition job on the four and five, now hit the bend running a close third. He was big and classy, knew the corner well, got halfway round and like a cyclist in a velodrome, cut down to the rails for that slingshot burst of speed. Once again he managed to totally obliterate the competition, this time the two and the three dogs, in so doing. Billy arrived on the scene as they were starting to get untangled. He, too, after so many circuits of the course knew just where the best route lay. Suddenly they're out of the corner, he's dived for the rails, and he's running third.

In Billy's distance racing heyday the last 300 metres were his and his alone. No dog around could match that withering finish. Ah, but all that was a good fifteen months ago, and this was a sprint. But suddenly Billy *was* sprinting! Halfway down the straight the old fella ranged up to the seven dog, waited his chance and in two strides slipped underneath him. Now he's second. There's 70 metres to go and the leader is at least five lengths clear. To a lesser dog, an impossible task, but great dogs don't think that way. This is the stuff that separates the great from the good and the super from the great. With every stride that ageing black canine collection of power and stamina gained on the tearaway leader. First a foot, then two. Then a length, then two. The post was too close, the task seemed impossible. But some dogs never give up. They have that incredible will to win. They know instinctively where the finish is: that invisible line stretching from one side of the track to the other. Billy knew and now it was only 20 metres away. Three lengths, two and a half, one and a half, he's on the leader's rump, no more than four strides to the line, and inexplicably the leader stumbles. Just a false stride, an infinitesimal moment in time, a metre from the post, but just enough. They cross the line as one. Billy on the inside, the red rug on the outer. Photo!

The bookies are betting on the result. I can only hope we've won it. The commentator can't separate them. The judge takes three minutes.

Sid gave me the print. It's faded now but carefully locked away with all those special treasures, collected and sometimes mused over when life allows time for reflection. Just a blurred picture of a dog. A greyhound that went from a very good dog to a super dog in the space of 200 metres. A dog with a heart so damn big that just three beats would drain Sydney Harbour. With a will to win like very few before or since. A stride from the lines and he loses, a stride or two past and he loses, but where it counts you can still make out a long thin greying muzzle straining with every ounce of determination, lunging for the line he knew was there, and getting to it in front, by no more than two centimetres!

Billy went on to win several more country races, but would contest no more in the city. In another six weeks he would injure the other leg in similar fashion and would be retired, living the rest of his days as Sid's pet.

Billy was a pioneer, he proved that surgical repair of muscle tears could work. On a lesser dog it may not have been so successful. Sid has passed from this mortal abode, and if heaven includes the odd greyhound then I know he'll find happiness.

Oh, yes, I nearly forgot. What about the 'Just once around tonight'? Well, it turned out that that's all Sid kept saying to the dog for the whole week leading up to the start, and 'You know, son,' he told me, 'I don't think the old fella listened till we got to those damn boxes. He looks at me as if to say, "What are we doing here, this is the wrong lot?" It's then that he understands. He knows what I mean about just once around. Should've saved me damn breath, shouldn't I?' Who knows, there's only one who does – and Billy's not telling.

3

The Cutlery

It's very hard when you're the junior of the practice and the boss sends you out on an errand that quite frankly he'd rather not perform. This was one of those days.

In and around Sydney there were large numbers of spelling properties, places where horses go to have a rest in between racing campaigns. Many of these were up in the Hills district north-west of suburbia – although these days, some thirty years on, most have been swallowed up by housing. The majority were around twenty or thirty acres and run by experienced horsemen, fellas with very little formal education, but who had a real bush knowledge and love of the equine animal. Dural is a pretty area, and Lightning Lodge was set on the side of a large shallow valley. It was home to well over twenty horses. Spelling in various yards would be everything from yearlings yet to see the white rails of a racecourse or feel a saddle and jockey on their back, right through to ageing campaigners resting their aching joints in the hope that Mother Nature would grant them just one more crack at the big time.

Charlie ran the place. 'Gotta bit of a problem with this gelding,' he said as we walked over to the stable area. There in a small yard stood a very haggard-looking brown horse. Not well grown by any standard, somewhat underweight and looking decidedly unwell.

'Hasn't touched an ounce of feed for the last two days.'

That was pretty obvious, the bin was overflowing and the hayrack likewise; the horse just stood there, head down, occasionally turning to cast a glance at his flanks.

'What's the story, Chasa?'

'Oh, this other bloke come here in a bit of a hurry the other day and he's gelded him all too quick for my liking.' I took it all in and shook down the thermometer to take the poor animal's temperature.

'Geez, he feels on fire,' and indeed he was, all of 2 degrees centigrade above normal in temperature. Even as we stood there I could feel him sweat.

'Did he drop him, or do him standing?' I asked.

'Left him standing, he did; don't like it, you know, much rather put 'em on the ground, they get up good and quiet that way.' Quite honestly, I prefer that too. Standing castrations are more than a little dangerous to a horse, not to mention the vet doing the job.

Infections following castration are not the norm. If everything goes smoothly, the whole wound should be completely healed within ten to fourteen days. But when infection does get a hold it can mean major resurgery or prolonged use of antibiotics.

'I'm hitting him with twenty mils of penicillin now and I'll leave you the bottle. Hit him with another fifteen every day.'

Sometimes something tells you just to have another look.

'Better just check out the wound before I go. Don't reckon he'll stand any sedation – can you twitch him for me?'

'No worries, H, you can rely on me.' And that I could. An experienced horseman on the head of a horse gives you the confidence to do most things to your patient. Gingerly I snaked a hand along the horse's abdomen and up towards the wound.

He flinched and kicked a little with the nearside hind, but eventually I got a couple of fingers inside.

'Guess what I've found?' I said as my thumb and finger closed on a familiar instrument. A quick squeeze and the ratchet released and out came a pair of clamps.

'Hang on again, I think there's another one.' And sure enough, there was. I now had both pairs in my left hand.

'Well,' said Chasa, 'the mongrel was in so much of a hurry to get out of the place he left the bloody cutlery behind.'

No wonder the horse was in so much trouble! It's customary to whip the clamps off some ten minutes or so after you've finished. They're just there for insurance in case something goes wrong. I know who the other bloke was. So does Chasa, and even to this day he brags about the couple of bits of cutlery he's got hangin' on the wall, ''cos that mongrel ain't comin' back here no more'.

4

Watching like a Hawk

Although it's well over thirty years since my days as a young vet in England, memories keep flooding back. It was a great place to work back then, although the money was pretty pathetic. My weekly salary was forty-nine guineas: let me translate that into real money. A guinea was one pound one shilling. It was used by the upper classes and pseudo-upper classes (like veterinarians) as a form of currency, although no such note ever existed. In other words, it was a bit toffy to talk in guineas rather than quids (pounds sterling). Back in those days one Aussie dollar would buy one English pound, so in real terms I was earning about fifty-four dollars a week – haven't things changed since then? Today it would take three Aussie dollars to buy the same English pound and the wages are now around 100 pounds a day. Does that mean the Poms are three times better than we are, or are we only a third as good as we used to be? Interesting question, eh, have you ever thought about that?

Out-of-hours work in an English winter is not much fun. It's cold enough during the daytime to freeze the washing on the clothesline, and without even the hint of sunshine, working on a frigid night is the pits.

'Is that you, vetinary?' garbled the Wiltshire farmer on the end of a crackling telephone line.

'Yes, it's me,' I retorted, waking almost automatically from total slumber to complete consciousness in the space of a millisecond. Vets are good at this and my wife has often wondered how in no time at all I can be instantly lucid and able to solve most veterinary problems in a twinkling and yet the light globe in the bathroom remains unreplaced some two weeks after it blew.

'I've got this sow.'

'Yes, what's wrong with the sow?'

'Well, sir . . . I think she's having trouble piggin.' A simple translation of which is, she's having a litter and something's gone wrong.

'Where do you live?' I queried, reaching for a pencil to scribble down an address.

'You been 'ere before, sire, you 'ave, it's down the Fordingbridge road about two miles past the Bull's Head just on the right, sir, I'll leave a light on for yer, sir.'

'I've gotta go, dunno when I'll be back, probably an hour or two, see you in the morning.' Vets' wives get used to this sort of life, vets are born to it.

A quick glance at the clock, it's 1.00 a.m. and pitch black outside. I've got enough layers of clothing on to withstand an Arctic blizzard. The Ford Anglia coughs, shudders and the motor springs to life. Heading off down the narrow road there's plenty of time to think, the only landscape in view is that illuminated by the headlights of the car stabbing their way through the enshrouding blackness of a Wiltshire night.

There's the place and sure enough the light's on, he's even got a cuppa tea in his hands – yeah, but not for me.

'Righto, where's this pig then?' Strike me, I'm even starting to sound like a Pom and I've only lived in the area five months.

With a tilly lantern swinging from his left hand he led the

way. We trudged through the mud and slush that is so much a part of any English farm in the winter, to the lopsided barn and this poor wretched sow. It wasn't much of a shed by Australian terms, more of a lean-to, lean being the operative word, but he was proud of it.

'My grandfather built this 'ere baarn.' Yeah, and poor old grandad never had a spirit level, I'll bet. Inside it was no warmer than outside. The wooden slats sheeting the building left gaping holes through which the northern winter crept with great dexterity. The floor was earthen and there was a central laneway with half a dozen crudely fashioned wooden pens on each side – most contained a sow, either suckling or about to farrow a litter.

The door on the pen swung open, it was only waist high and seemed such a flimsy structure to hold such a huge animal. Sows are big. Very, very big! And very, very strong! This old girl lay on her side on a thick bed of warm barley straw. She was what we'd call a large white landrace cross, a mountain of a mother with eight greedy youngsters reefing and tugging at the double row of nipples. An infra-red light and reflector hung over the assembly.

'Well, what's worrying you?' I said.

'I don't think she be finished, sir,' he said. Only one thing for it and that's to go in and have a look. Off with half the clothes, on with the overalls. Roll up the right sleeve, pull on the long rubber glove. There were no such things as throwaway plastic gloves in those days. You looked after your long rubber glove like a long-lost friend. Washed it thoroughly after every use, dried it carefully and then doused the whole thing with a liberal layer of talcum powder to prevent it perishing, before returning it to the little green tin that was its home. Yeah, I've still got the little green tin and the powder, but the glove has seen better days. It's one of those stupid little souvenirs that you wonder why you ever bothered keeping, but you do. Ah, if only that little tin could talk, there are plenty of memories trapped inside. Good idea – I'll check it out and share a few more with you after I finish this story.

Sorry, I got distracted. Now I'm kneeling behind the old girl and applying a good dollop of lubricant to the glove encasing my right arm.

'This be 'er first litter, sir . . . aye, this be 'er first. She been strainin' real 'ard fer must be nigh on two 'ours when I be ringin' yer.' Armed with this valuable piece of information I joined the pig on the straw and introduced my right arm into the only area of warmth in the entire building, the inside of a pig. I like pigs, they're great animals and really clean if given half a chance. The sow didn't seem to mind my intrusions, but continued to strain as my arm slid slowly up one horn of her uterus. Sorry, gang, but we need to divert again for a quick anatomy lesson. Sows have big litters, twelve or fourteen is the norm for a mature female. The uterus is shaped like the letter 'Y' – the vertical part we call the body and the two arms we call the horns. A pig's uterus has a small body and very lengthy horns, and they need them to accommodate all those piglets.

We have a saying, 'Farrowing a sow is like pulling on an overcoat with a six-foot sleeve.' There I am buried up to the armpit inside this pig, literally pulling each horn of the uterus up over my gloved arm like the aforementioned distorted overcoat. It seems to go on forever. Finally I get to the end of one horn.

'Nothing left in there.'

'Aye, sir . . . but she be strainin' . . . I'd not gotcha out 'ere, sir, if she not be strainin' . . . rrr [a favourite Wiltshire expression with which an entire conversation can be conducted] . . . me auld dad, sir . . . 'im be havin' a lot of pigs, sir . . . rrr . . . 'e be knowin' she be in trouble, sir, that's why I be callin' yer.'

OK, fair enough, there must be one left on the other side.

Here I go again, pulling on the overcoat in a strictly metaphorical sense, because everything is so slippery that I can't get a grip and the sow's straining as well, so the muscle in my upper arm feels like someone's applying a tourniquet. At last I can touch it, feel a foot, but can't quite grab it, everything is just too slippery. For twenty minutes my right hand gropes and strains to grasp the tiny hoof and drag the hapless piglet into the world. No way, I know when I'm beaten.

'She'll have to have a Caesarean to get it out,' I explained.

'Yes, sir, you be the boss, sir, . . . rrr . . . me auld dad 'e 'ad to 'ave an operation 'is self just last week otherwise 'e be 'ere 'elpin' the two of us.' God forbid!

'Now I'm gonna have to duck back to the clinic to get a bit of gear, you stay here and keep an eye on things. Don't leave her on her own, OK?'

'Rrr . . . you be right with me, sir . . . I be watchin' 'er like a 'awk.'

Forty minutes later the pig's lolling off to sleep and I'm getting ready to open things up and pull out the remaining piglet. It's a pretty simple piece of surgery done under less than hospital-like conditions; the main object of the exercise is to incise through the flank of the sow, locate the offending youngster, cut it free of the uterus and sew the whole lot up again. All this while keeping the farmer's hands, and the half a bale of straw on which I'm kneeling to perform the procedure, out of the wound. Time to get on with things. The scalpel flashes down the sterilised pink skin, my able assistant is being anything but that, standing almost over the top of me as I grope inside the uterus. His head is almost alongside mine, desperate to take in the full surgical scene complete with blood and entrails. He's even breathing all over me as I grope around inside the uterus and pull out the first horn.

'This side's empty.'

'Rrr . . . must be in the other side, sir.' Geez, his breath stinks . . . Not halitosis, but something a little more sinister, I fear. So in we go again. Grab the other horn and haul it out into full view.

'Rrr . . . There be nothin' in that one either, sir.' He was right, how embarrassing. I'd chopped this pig open to pull out one lousy piglet at three o'clock in the morning and it's just not there.

'Rrr . . . where it be, sir . . . where it be?'

'Buggered if I know . . . just shut up and let me get on with it.'

'Rrr . . . don't be gettin' upset now, vetinary.' I was. What a waste of time. I reefed the last couple of stitches up tight and cleaned down the wound. I was going to get to the bottom of this if it killed me – I counted the piglets again, still the same eight happy little souls. Where in heaven's name had number nine gone?

My farming friend was standing well back now, scratching a whiskery chin with the gnarled fingers of his right hand, a ridiculous hand-knitted beanie pulled down tightly over both ears.

'Rrr . . . she be a real mystery then . . . eh? You sure she 'ad another young 'un in 'er belly?' Of course I was bloody sure.

'Come over here and give me a hand. Let's just pull her out away from the wall.'

And it took all our strength to move my patient from one laying position to another.

'Rrr . . . well, sir, will you be lookin' at that then, there be the other little fella, she be layin' on 'im and squashin' 'im flat.' He was dead right, as right as the piglet was dead. The question was, how did the piglet get from the inside to the outside without anyone noticing?

'I asked you to keep a watch on her the whole time, what happened?' I angrily enquired.

'I did, sir, . . . I did . . . rrr . . . I only be goin' up t' 'ouse for a little somethin' to keep out t' chill.' And it wasn't the beanie he was talking about. There, its thin brown neck snaking out of the right pocket of his overcoat, was a large bottle of brandy. The old fella was half-shot. I could read between the lines: it was a bit cold down in the piggery and a bit warmer up at the house. It was only a pig. She'd been trying for two hours. Nothing was going to happen in the forty minutes I was away, so he'd keep himself warm on the inside with a dram or two of the alcoholic stuff and on the outside in an armchair close to the fire.

So what's the lesson in all of this? Never take the word of a Wiltshire pig farmer whose every conversation begins with 'rrr'.

5

The Little Green Tin

You carry all sorts of equipment when you're a country vet. Patients can include anything from the family pet budgie right through to a massive draughthorse stallion and everything in between, although there was only so much you could fit in the boot of the Anglia.

I probably should take a moment to describe the vehicle. Essentially it was about the most unstable car I've ever tried to drive. The centre of gravity was probably somewhere about head height and on every corner the car would lurch and roll almost uncontrollably. It was built totally out of proportion, measuring more in height than in length or width. Fully manual gearbox with overdrive top gear, about as much guts as a bicycle and wouldn't pull the skin off a rice custard – but it was the practice car, it was cheap to run and every other vet had pranged it except me. (Mind you, I managed to maintain the record with a head-on into a Morris Minor just a week before the job finished.) The seats were as hard as rocks, the steering wheel thin and slippery and the back seat had a bad habit of disengaging itself, allowing the contents of the boot to spill over into the back of the car.

We carried ropes and chains, not for the car, but for calving cows. There were boxes of drugs, cartons of bottles, bags of instruments, both large and small, and copious quantities of iodine and saline solution. The practice mainly looked after dairy cattle. Massive Friesian Holsteins (the big black and white ones to you guys) who suffered from 'loo', the Wiltshire term for 'foul of the foot'. Time to explain.

The Salisbury Plain is home to many great landmarks, the most remarkable of which, in my opinion, is Stonehenge. Almost daily my calls would take me past this most incredible of all ancient monuments. To hear the wind whine and sigh around the great stone circle and to feel the warmth of the summer sun on the rocks as afternoon became twilight gave the place a special something, to me. How and why was it built, no one really seems to know, but it has some magnetic force which pervades your very insides. I feel privileged to have known it as it was in those days, not as it is today, hemmed in by barbed wire and security guards.

The countryside grows great grass, probably because the soil lies over large masses of limestone. Chunks of this rock have metamorphosed through volcanic activity into hard flint. Much of the housing utilises this material in its construction. Typically the stone is interwoven with bright orange brickwork but each village seemed to have its own particular building style. Early man, who probably built so many circles like Stonehenge, used the flint for other purposes. When the stones are broken into smaller pieces each fragment has at least one very sharp edge. Our ancients used these as tools of trade and early cutting instruments.

The problem for modern dairy cows was simply this. The pastures were strewn with thousands of these naturally occurring sharp fragments of flint, which would find their way up between the two toes of any foot and cause immense pain, infection and lameness. Half our days in practice were spent removing these wretched foreign objects from the struggling hooves of less than cooperative cows. Facilities were poor; there were none of your modern steel piping yards, it was an old wooden stockrace held together with wire and baling twine or a portable bail set up somewhere in the middle of a paddock. It required patience, physical strength and sometimes a bit of luck to locate the offending fragment in a hurry.

Not every dairy was quite this primitive. There were a few quite modern farmers in and around the district – men who'd discovered that concrete really did make life a lot easier and that a herringbone bail got milking done much more quickly than the old-fashioned single walk-through situation.

Ernest was a young bloke, he'd inherited the farm from his dad, who was now crippled with agonising rheumatoid arthritis. A top bloke, around my age, happy to listen to suggestions and always interested in how similar farmers were doing things in other countries. He read a lot and made sweeping changes to the way in which the old property functioned. There was a central laneway to make bringing in cattle a simple routine. The dairy itself was one of the first herringbones in the district. Not big by today's standards, but he could milk eight a side almost on his own.

So what's a herringbone? To most of the farmers around it was quite a revolution. Viewed from above, the reason for the name becomes obvious. The central axis is a pit some five feet deep and about the same in width. The cows walk in on both sides and stand at an angle of about 45 degrees to the pit with their udders and hindquarters at about face level and their heads buried in the feed bins that run along both of the internal walls. All the milking equipment hangs from the roof overhead and it is simply a matter of washing the udder, drying the excess and applying the milking cups.

There's only one drawback with a herringbone, in my view. Two excretory orifices are at the same end as the udder. The operator needs to wear an apron and some headgear or risk getting showered with either urine or manure. Or else, you need very well-trained cows.

Because the farm ran so smoothly, it was not often that veterinary attention was needed. It had probably been at least nine or ten weeks since I'd last paid a call. Mind you, Ern and I were about the same age and inclined to enjoy a pint at The Haunch in town every so often. He loved to ask me all about Australia.

The two-way crackled into life and the squeaky voice of the practice receptionist broke the silence. 'Base to car two . . . base to car two.'

'Car two receiving, over,' I replied with the microphone held close to my lips.

'Harry, there's a cow to clean on the Bournemouth road, you know the Stephens place.' I did.

'OK, I'll be there in about half an hour.'

Cleaning cows is a shorthand description for a fairly unpleasant sort of procedure. Quite often after calving the cow fails to pass the afterbirth with the calf. It simply remains stuck inside. Lots of problems can ensue, the main one being infection, within the uterus itself and almost invariably the udder becomes affected as well due to the rotting material dragging along behind the cow as she walks. It's not a job for the faint-hearted. Even talking about it brings back memories of that terrible smell. Who'd marry a vet?

'I've got her in for you, Harry,' Ern greeted my arrival with eager anticipation.

'Geez, you've done a bit around here, old son, since my last visit.'

'Yes, Harry, I've been anxious to tidy up around the parlour [that's English farming talk for bails], get rid of all the muck and slush about the place.' He'd done a good job too and we talked of other things as the little green tin sprang open and the long rubber glove slid up my right arm. Boy, what a rotten job, in your face, up your nose, it's so close to the origin of the horrid stench. It took me a good ten minutes to loosen most of the offending material and pull it free, but there was still a remnant or two that just wouldn't come.

'I'm just gonna duck back to the Anglia and get a couple of these new whiz-bang foaming pessaries.'

'They are really good, are they, Harry?' Ern asked so politely.

'Yeah, mate, just the go for problems like this. We'll pop a couple of them inside, they foam up just like a bubble bath and shift all the muck around the place.'

'By golly, Harry, they do sound just the shot.' Ern was so much more cultured than the average Wiltshire farmer.

'I'll be back in a flash.' And I headed off around the corner of the herringbone shed. Funny, I thought for just a second I heard Ern call my name. No, must have imagined it. Turning back towards the yards I saw he was waving. I waved back, turned the corner and strode feet first and neck deep into his latest addition . . . Yes, folks, the slurry pit. Liquid shit, dairy manure, recycled grass, call it whatever you like, I was standing in it up to my chin and there's Ern, red-faced and apologising profusely while extending a right hand to help pull me out.

'I'm terribly sorry, Harry . . . terribly sorry.'

'Where are the bloody steps?'

'Oh, you're so right, Harry, another design fault – there aren't any steps.'

'And there's no bloody fence or cover over the top of it either!' I spluttered as we both dragged my soggy form from the semi-liquid sludge.

So we cleaned the cow with my whiz-bang foaming pessaries, he cleaned me with the wash-down hose from the dairy and we both went inside for a clothing change (yes, you always carry a spare set of everything) and the customary afternoon tea which his mother insisted I stay for. She was a damned good cook and the scones and homemade blackberry jam were to die for.

Only one drawback to the whole event, a man couldn't walk into The Haunch for a quiet ale any more without the whole bar making some stupid remark about 'watching where you walk' and 'How's the swimming going, what sort of stroke do you use these days?'

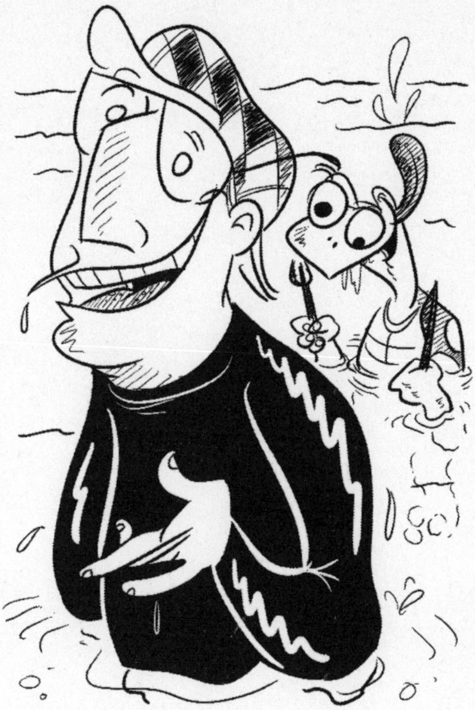

Talking with the Animals Again

6

In Turtle Soup

As far as television programs go, 'Talk to the Animals' had a pretty good run. Four years with an annual output of 40 shows is a hefty 160 episodes. As the end drew near, the Seven Network was trialling a news service which went to air each evening at 5.00 p.m., in direct opposition to Channel Ten. The experiment proved unsuccessful and with the withdrawal of the early bulletin something had to be found to take its place. That something was 'Talk to the Animals' – not as a regular one-hour episode, but rather as a very much shortened, 'best of', if you like, half-hour show.

The amount of work involved in putting this sort of series to air is immense. There is all the researching through hours and hours of previous episodes, looking for the very best of what had been aired over the last four years. Then it was a matter of arranging, softening, editing and occasionally modifying those existing stories to make them fit one with another and into the half-hour format. It was my job as host of the original 160 episodes to also introduce this new format and to link the stories so the whole thing flowed evenly and smoothly along.

The job involved simply (and I use the word somewhat loosely in this context), facing the camera and talking about some animal that was near at hand, while 'throwing' – a term we use to mean introducing the next anecdote and its presenter.

For obvious reasons, the whole job had to be accomplished both quickly and cheaply, and with that in mind I often found myself at zoos, farms, aquariums and the like, where a whole gaggle of species were on hand to choose from.

'Harry, you'd better put this wetsuit on, mate,' the curator of the marine pool at the entrance to Manly Aquarium advised.

'It's not that cold,' I remarked, feeling quite at home in the warmer climes of Sydney after some six or more years in Tassie.

'Take it from me, mate, you'll need it.' You don't argue with the experts, this was his domain, mine was very much on dry land. Getting into a wetsuit for the first time I must have looked like some tortured black crab, pulling and struggling with the seemingly endless rubber tubes that make up the arms and legs. Eventually the thing was zipped up.

'I should get in there with him,' the curator advised my producer.

'No, mate . . . we just want Harry in there . . . he'll be right . . . won't you, mate?'

Heaven knows why I nodded a 'yes'.

Over the side and into the pool. It's around four and a half feet deep, a metre and a half to the metrically minded, and filled with all these gorgeous turtles. Two or three different species swam lazily around in the warm, clear water. One or two were extremely large with shells nearly a metre across. It wasn't their shells that caught my attention, but rather their mouths. The majority had jaws like a parrot's. Huge beaks that opened and closed regularly as they swam.

'Harry. A piece of advice, mate . . . don't stand still, just keep walking around, will ya?' my instructor in all things turtle-like advised, in a low voice. So the dance began. With a slow walking, or was it waltzing, motion the 'TV vet bloke' in the black wetsuit was off.

'For God's sake, Harry, will you keep still?' yells Kevin, my friend and producer. 'The damn soundo can't hear a word you're saying when you get to the back of the pond. Come down the front and damn well stand still.' Not a sign of my backstop, the curator. Better do as I'm told.

'Stand over here, mate, you'll be right. Look relaxed. OK. Now sort of lean over the front of the pond and look up at the camera. That's great; OK, H, go for it.'

'G'day, welcome to another episode of 'Talk to the Animals'. I'm at Manly Aquarium in the turtle pool. There are some fascinating animals that inhabit the warmer waters of the Australian coast and some of the Pacific islands nearby – yyyyyyyyyyyyyyy!' and I was out of that tank like a shot. My left hand at the same time darted round to the left side of my rear end to find a gaping hole, not only in the wetsuit, but in the swimmers and in me as well! Hell! Can these things bite! Swimming lazily around the pond was a huge snapping turtle with a mouthful of my wetsuit and a sample of my swimming trunks firmly grasped in that huge, bony beak.

Dave the curator arrives nonchalantly back on the scene.

'Told you they bite, Harry,' he observes, surveying the aquatic disaster.

'What if we feed them?' asks Kev, ever keen to get that perfect shot.

'You really do want them to eat Harry, don't you?' Dave exclaims. 'Let him get back in again, but don't let him stop. Once they get the taste of something they come back for more.'

I hoped he was kidding. So what started off as a slow waltz rapidly turned into a three-step and ended as full-scale rock 'n' roll, as the turtles and I fairly streaked around that pool.

Delivering lines to a camera while keeping one eye out for that ferocious beak takes some doing.

'That's why we always wear wet suits,' observes Dave ever so casually as I struggle out of what's left of this one and head for the shark tank.

'No, mate – I am not getting in with those.' Kev just nods.

7

Horses for Courses

Singapore was a regular overseas stopover for 'Talk to the Animals'. In all, there were three trips, the last being without a doubt the most uncomfortable and the most memorable.

International Racehorse Transport was a company that specialised in doing exactly what its name suggested. Transporting horses from one part of the globe to another. We were to accompany one of these shipments from Australia to Singapore. There are large numbers of young thoroughbreds in Australia that simply fail to make the grade as top line racehorses; in fact, the likelihood of picking a successful horse when it's a youngster at the yearling sales is only average. 'Breed the best, feed the best, buy the best and hope for the best' – that's the way it goes. Many of the two-year-olds that fail to make it even as country prospects can often find markets overseas, where the standard is not as high as our own and where gambling is truly a way of life. Hence Singapore and Malaysia are often looked upon as the places to purchase such horses. They must have at least raced and preferably placed on a track somewhere, be under the age of three and be sound.

The whole procedure starts with the purchase of the horses through a livestock agent in Australia acting for clients in Asia. These are often businessmen, or in some cases the trainers themselves. Having been selected and paid for, the horses are then identified by brands and often by DNA typing. They undergo a period of quarantine at racing stables and a thorough veterinary examination to ensure they are free from any serious injury before the sale is completed. Then it's just a matter of waiting out the quarantine period, getting the paperwork in order and ensuring their transport is organised.

These horses have seen many a horse float in their time and load easily into the trucks that will take them to the airport. Through special security and heavy screening the trucks drive onto the tarmac. The camera crew and I have followed every step of the journey. As the thoroughbreds step down from the relative safety of the transporter, they have about them almost a sense of expectancy, and a touch of uneasiness. Gone are the familiar surroundings of trees and stables, tracks and yards. Nothing here now except acres of concrete, scorching hot in the late spring sun. Their handlers have been through this a hundred times before. With hands and with words they calm their anxious animals. From now until we land in Singapore their home will be the sky stalls which at the moment sit on the tarmac, atop a string of trailers. Each is just big enough for one horse. In design they are very much the same as a starting stall, but there is no way out the front. Four horses fit each cluster of stalls. Without hesitation all but a nervous chestnut filly simply walk up the ramp, into the stall and the gates are locked behind.

In the front of each cluster is a narrow passageway. Through here we feed and water the horses on the trip. Lush biscuits of lucerne are squeezed inside brand-new hay nets and hung just inside the front of each stall. 'The green tranquilliser, we call it,' says Pauline, a carer on so many trips. Her soothing way of talking, her gentle but firm way of getting the horse to do what she wants, are legendary in the industry. It's a special gift some people have. A gift of talking to horses. A gift of understanding them, and a gift of being able to exercise control when necessary.

The chestnut filly is starting to turn it on a bit. There's always the worry that she'll stir the others up and then we will have problems. Crispin reaches inside his bulging case for a small bottle of tranquilliser. He draws up about 3 ml. He has trouble with the vein. I offer my services and steadily the yellow drug snakes into the filly's jugular vein. No more than ten minutes later we are leading and lifting the filly into her box. With arms locked behind, Crispin and I lift while Pauline on the head urges her to step up and into her temporary home. She's in. The gates lock behind. In another moment she finds the lucerne and begins to eat. Everyone breathes a sigh of relief.

Waiting seems to take an eternity, but eventually we are on our way over to the plane, the little tractor pulling its load of twelve young thoroughbreds, none of whom seem to be giving two hoots about the trip so far. Even the filly is as good as gold. A reversal of horsepower, I think, but then that's the way it is today. Horses are for pleasure, not for work any more.

The giant scissors backed their way under each unit of four stalls and ever so slowly lifted the huge container up level with the floor of the cargo hold. From here a series of rollers allowed the sky stalls to be manoeuvred into position. I rode up with the last four. We were in the tail end of a 747 combi, a jumbo whose rear one-third was taken up with cargo. Up front the passengers had not the slightest idea what was behind the bulkhead at the rear of their cabin. Straps from every side and every angle secured the stalls in place. The floor grid was locked. Everything was secure. Guess what? We were sharing the trip with two and a half tons of broccoli. All neatly packed in white polystyrene cartons and smothered in ice to keep it fresh. The horses seemed totally unmoved.

For take-off the crew and I are seated in the last row of the cabin. The flight is full, but no one seems to notice our constant comings and goings as we track back and forth between our thoroughbred cargo and our seats. The cargo compartment is huge. None of your fancy trim in here, just bare aluminium structure and external skin. Wires, there are literally kilometres of wires running back and forth across the walls of the hold. The floor is dangerous. It's flat with a whole series of roller balls fitted just above flush to allow for easy manoeuvring of crates and containers, but it's very hard to walk on.

'Keep to the sides when you're in there,' advises Crispin. 'If we get any turbulence there's something to hang on to.'

So far everything has gone to plan. There's little more than an hour to go. All the horses have travelled well. Each has drunk plenty. Dehydration is an even bigger problem for animals when flying than it is for us humans.

Then it hits. We are in the middle of a tropical storm. The plane plunges 300 feet in three seconds. All of us grab for the nets that cover the broccoli and the walls, hanging on to anything that might be secure. All except our trusty producer. Len is into his imitation of a drunken crab. Slithering all over the floor, unable to get any sort of a grip with his Reeboks. Now he's into a copy of Roy and H.G.'s 'Hello, boys'. The harder he tries to grab the wall, the more spreadeagled he becomes. The only ones not laughing are Len and the horses.

Poor devil, it took him a good minute of crawling on his hands and knees before he reached the safety of the nets. He was always a trifle red-faced. He was a lot more so now.

Touchdown in Singapore and of course it's raining and late at night. Rosie the cameraman is cursing the lack of light and the wet weather, Andy the soundo is still laughing about 'the human spider in the cargo hold'. We get our shots, I say my little piece. The horses go off with their intended trainers to spend another two days in quarantine, before heading north to Malaysia, and we head off to the hotel for a good night's sleep. Tomorrow we will check on the horses, but by then Pauline and Crispin will be on their way back home to prepare for yet another shipment.

8

Singapore Birds

When 'TTTA' first began we were just a group of five. Two girls, Pam and Kelly; three blokes, Richard, Mike and myself. As time progressed the crew was strengthened with the addition of Steve and Jane, and then Tess replaced Pam when she left to marry. It was Kelly who joined us the next day in Singapore, all primed and ready to do a story on the Asian jungle fowl.

Now this might at first sound just a trifle boring but these birds are in fact the predecessors of many modern breeds of poultry, particularly the hard-feathered group, which comprises most of the magnificently coloured game birds. The birds live in what little jungle remains on some of the smaller islands outlying the coast of Singapore proper. This meant an early start and a ferry trip in a pretty dilapidated diesel-engined relic of a vessel to one such island. Here we were met by our guide.

He was a very well-spoken gentleman of Indian descent with a very adequate black beard, dark eyes and a physical build more reminiscent of a weight-lifter. He was also an avid conservationist. Kelly was instantly enraptured by his presence, never leaving his side for the whole of the day. Although the island was small, the trek across to our likely spotting point was both long and treacherous. First, a local taxi, disguised as a cancerous collection of rusting panels and flaking paint, with a motor so in need of a tune and an exhaust system so full of holes it's a matter of amazement that we made it without suffering terminal carbon monoxide poisoning. Then it was out of the car and into the jungle. Don't get the wrong idea, though, there was a well-defined path as this area attracted many ornithologists. Mind you, they would spend weeks there; we had three hours to find the elusive fowl.

'This looks a good spot for an interview,' suggests our illustrious producer, and with that, Kelly and our guide take up their positions astride a huge rotting log just off to one side of the path.

'H, you shut up.' It's hard to understand why I'm so often asked to do that. 'Just go for a wander or something but stay right out of shot.' That's OK. I don't need to be told twice. And so began what to this day Noel Jones reckons is the world's longest interview. If the camera tapes were of good quality you could expect around thirty-three minutes a tape. Kelly filled two! Every question carefully thought out and every answer slow and detailed, for our guide spoke almost in poetic language. Kelly was besotted, I reckon! So there's the host of the show, me, just sitting there bored totally out of existence, when suddenly behind the two of them I see the bird. It's walking slowly and gingerly along a tree branch, about five metres behind and a couple of metres above their heads. Surely the cameraman can see it. It must be in his peripheral vision (for most operators film with one eye open for something that might happen outside the viewfinder's range).

The bird's nearing the end of the branch as the discussion drags on. I tap the producer on the shoulder. 'Sit down, H.' I point excitedly to the tree branch gently swaying with the weight of the bird. 'Will you shut up, Harry?'

It's all too much. Two steps back, 'click' goes the telephoto lens as it snaps onto the trusty Pentax, up to the eye, the motor drive's 'schlack . . . schlack' speeds the Kodachrome 400 through the aperture. In an instant the bird's gone, flying directly over their heads and disappearing into the jungle on the other side of the pathway. A brilliant montage of reds and yellows, greens so dark they are all but black and long sickle feathers of the tail streaming behind him. A fully mature cock bird. Boy, what a sight.

'Did ya see it? Did ya see it?' I blurt out, unable to control my excitement.

'See what?' says Noel, looking up from the camera.

'The bird, the bird!'

'What bird?' interrupts the now rather annoyed producer.

'The jungle fowl. It flew right over your heads while the two of you were sitting there.'

Noel rewound the tape . . . no bird, he was too tight. Guess who got the shots? Full frame too, shame it wasn't on video!

The episode put something of a dampener on things as our guide restated that the birds were rare and to see another in this vicinity would be highly unlikely. So we did the only thing possible, trekked on to the local village. The chief was halfway pleased to see us. I don't think he cared too much for the opposite sex. Yes, he had such a bird as we needed in a cage, behind his none-too-elaborate house. Could we film the bird? Well, perhaps. First we must take tea with him. An elaborate ceremony that involved repeated pourings, stirrings and the addition of God knows what to the original brew in the pot. The stuff looked like kerosene, and tasted about the same.

Gesticulating at me through the multilayered sarong that draped awkwardly over his ageing frame, he indicated that it would only be me who would hold the bird (obviously one bird man can recognise another). This bird was a somewhat dishevelled replica of the magnificent specimen I'd captured with the Pentax earlier in the day. With a bit of trickery, Noel was able to make it seem that rather than being held tightly by the feet, the rare specimen was in fact moving slowly through the jungle. 'The camera never lies' – don't you believe it. Back went the bird into the cage. Much more ceremonial drinking of tea, and my stomach was in revolt. Surely it was time for lunch.

Back into our ramshackle taxi and we are bumping our way to the other side of the island and a feed of chilli crab. Just the thing for your bowels when you're far from home and a toilet. The restaurant was nothing flash, even by local standards. Just an assortment of steel collapsible tables and chairs, long wooden benches and rickety wooden stools, all under the protection of partially rotted canvas. The kitchen was definitely open-air. There was not enough canvas to stretch that far. The tucker smelt great. Anything to get rid of the petroleum taste would be sensational.

'Where's the toilet?' asks Kell in her modest female voice.

The guide is at pains to explain that the toilet available here is just a trifle out of left field. He points to a long jetty. A falling-down wooden structure extending some 150 metres out into the quiet waters of the bay. At the far end is what could quite rightly be described as an 'outhouse'. She's handed a toilet roll and departs.

A good ten minutes elapses. Kelly returns and the food is served.

'Boy, this tastes good,' announces Andy the soundo. Everyone else responds with vigorous nodding, their mouths stuffed with food.

'Where do you catch the crabs?' enquires Kell of our waiter. Unable to speak much English he deflects the question to the guide.

'Well,' he describes to Kell in whispered tones, 'the crabs are caught out in the bay. The fishermen set traps every day. They are a specialty of the area.'

'Do they catch them out near the jetty?' she enquires.

'Oh yes, definitely, the very best crabs are caught around the jetty.'

It was all too much. Kell went back and sat in the taxi. We finished our crabs. He was right about one thing, that guide of ours, these were the very best crabs.

9

Broome or Bust

Back in the 'TTTA' days we found ourselves in every corner of Australia as well as overseas, but before any trip could be undertaken, research had to be done. Tourist authorities both here and overseas are pretty aware of just how important it is that the right look and appeal of their neck of the woods be portrayed to the world at large. The tourist dollar even then was a mighty one. So it was armed with all the relevant information that Rosie, Andy, Steve and myself headed for the wilds of Western Australia. Our producer was the lady of repute from my last book. You've got it. Suzantasaurus. The big one, complete with briefcases chockers full of all the information she could muster. Unfortunately, most of it was wrong.

First port of call was Kununurra.

'Are we really going to fly in this little thing?' she stammered, as we scrambled aboard a small twin-engine aircraft. There is so much gear to carry around on these shoots, that on light aircraft we always book an extra seat just to allow for the weight of the equipment. After a couple of hours she was glad to get off.

'I really don't like flying. Can we get a real plane next time?'

'Sorry, lady, these are the only real planes we've got around here,' our pilot assured her.

There was one story for me here. A day with a flying vet who spends most of his days in the cockpit or on massive cattle stations, pregnancy testing (you know, what we vets call the old one-arm suntan routine, and, yes, I'm in there getting a tan too, while he's advising on farm management in general).

In the afternoon it's a visit to the local dairy farm for Steve. I went along for the ride, you can always pick up some useful info. The cattle were experimental crosses between native Indian milking cows and our own British breeds, like Friesians and Jerseys. These tropical cattle look so different with that huge hump sitting right on top of their shoulders and long bits of spare skin hanging down underneath like a theatre curtain. These are the hallmarks of the 'Bos indicus' breed, and they are very dominant in the crosses. But it is their resistance to tick-transmitted diseases, and their ability to handle the tropical monsoonal climate that makes them valuable. To increase quality and quantity of milk by cross-breeding them with traditional Australian dairy stock is the objective. The pastures grazed were so very different as well, grass grows almost a metre high and subtropical legumes twist their vine-like stems to the top of the sward. How different to the rye grass and clover of Tasmania. The days were hot, but humidity was low. The place was tolerable – that was, until we went to get a feed that night.

The motel didn't serve any meals and we were directed to one of the local pubs for some tucker. The big 'S' elected to stay in and do 'more research'.

Right away you got the feeling that this was a very cliquey town. Four total strangers walking into the local, we must have stood out like the horn on a unicorn. Buying a beer was no trouble, getting a feed – well, that's another story. An hour after ordering a simple steak, not one meal had turned up.

'Blow this, I'm starving. The meat's just sitting there – if the cook doesn't show up in a minute I'll hurdle the bar and cook it myself.'

'Steady on, H, there's more of them than us,' advises Rosie. He was right, there'd have been a free-for-all. But I did spark some action. The cook arrived on the scene. To say he seemed inebriated would be an understatement. This bloke was gone for all money. Couldn't even stand straight. Lurched in, put out a hand to steady his stride. 'Hissssss' right onto the hot plate. Muttering a few obscenities he threw the food onto the greasy steel cooktop and cremated our meals, swigging from a half-empty can of the 'green stuff' (VB) as he did. That's one place I'll never go back to, Ord River or no Ord River.

Broome was a coastal town and our accommodation something fantastic, right on the famous Cable Beach with its kilometres of sand, its camel rides and horse trekking. Right from the start this joint had a good feel. Honeymooners were everywhere around the resort. Seemed strange for four blokes to be there pretty well on our own. The big 'S' kept to herself. Steve had a couple of stories to do. One on bird migration that involved trapping numerous small birds with a mist net in the early hours of the morning, identifying them by species, tagging and releasing. He reckoned the mossies out there were bigger than the birds!

The major story of the whole trip was to be a visit to an Aboriginal settlement up the coast a bit. This community was believed to have a very close association with native fauna in their area. The big 'S' was so excited, fear of flying was thrown to the wind as the little Cessna careered down the runway and up into the sky. It was a magnificent day. We flew at low altitude all along the coast.

'What are you lot doin' up 'ere?' He was the dead spit of

Chips Rafferty. Right out of the 1940s. Six foot something tall, gaunt and heavily tanned, a big broad-brimmed Akubra angled slightly to the side, and driving a battered old Toyota troop carrier. Between us we loaded most of the gear into the back of the jalopy.

'We've come here to see the turtles, the fish and the sea eagle,' I replied quite excitedly.

'You're wastin' yer bloody time then, aren't ya?'

'Why?' I whispered, somewhat taken aback by his attitude.

'Well, they eat the turtles, poison the fish, and the bird hasn't been back for months. Reckon some mongrel must have shot it.' Wow.

'Rosie . . . better come over and have a listen to this.'

My newfound friend repeated the sentence for Rosie's benefit.

'Geez, mate, that doesn't leave us too much to shoot does it?'

It didn't. The big 'S' was summoned.

'I had no idea,' she stammered.

'Well, what are we going to do?' demanded an exasperated cameraman.

'Oh well, we'll have a little meeting.' We always had a little meeting when the big 'S' was floundering.

The local elder and some of the younger community members decided that as all of the above was true and correct we should just shoot some scenery and depart. But then, there was that bird colony on another island, and, hang on a minute, the kids could do a corroboree dance. Problem was, we couldn't get one of the dancers out of his Billabong tracksuit.

Steve was not to be denied, he wanted an interview with the elder at least.

'Legend has it,' he began, 'that your tribe would ride on these turtles and that you could get safely back to shore if a shark attacked you.'

'Dat mide've bin all right in dem days,' he said, 'but today de guvenment, him give us dem aluminium boats and safety jacket tings . . . we don't need dem no more.' Wow. We were going nowhere fast, until a well-spoken young man turned up. He was fairly senior in the group and did take us on an interesting trip to a couple of the smaller islands and could report on the history. But let's face it, there were no pictures worth taking – everything we had come to see was dead! So much for research . . . wait till the office hears about this!

Our pilot gave us a complimentary tour of the horizontal falls up north. It's a fascinating phenomenon. Imagine a chain of long, narrow islands, almost touching one another, set about half a kilometre from shore. The tide changes are so rapid and so massive that the water on the ocean side of these thin stretches of land is either dramatically higher or lower than the water between them and the coast. The rush of water between the two areas is funnelled through a narrow gap separating the two largest islands. The effect is to create a waterfall with water in massive volumes cascading down an imaginary cliff strung across the space between. An incredible sight.

Back at the resort, yours truly made for the phone to let the bosses of the outfit know just what a total waste of time and money the whole exercise had been. Guess what. The phone was engaged. Big 'S' had beaten me to it. After that, I must confess, the four of us held a council of war. We would do the rest of this trip without her and to hell with the consequences. This was mutiny in Broome, but at least we would go home with some stories.

That's how I came to meet up with Malcolm Douglas and his crocodile farm. A story we were told not to do because it was too politically sensitive. What a lot of garbage. Top bloke. A hunter turned conservationist, and boy, did he have some big brutes on hand. The breeding facility was fascinating, though even the newly hatched young had razor-sharp teeth and a cry like something out of Jurassic Park that had every female croc in the park on full alert. I've written of Malcolm elsewhere.

Over dinner that night the talk was of how to fill in the last day. The story set down for me was a no-go, once again through poor research. The animals had long left the area. Our hostess for the night suggested a visit to their local cattle station. Cath worked at night running the resort and managed to get back to the station about twice a week. She would be happy to drive us out there, but it'd be an early start.

The Land Rover handled the two-hour trip with ease, and we piled out into the arid, austere countryside. The air feels so dry and yet so clean in your nostrils, it's like no other place on earth.

'We'll move and muster a few head for you around the homestead if you'd like,' Cath advised, and Rosie set up for some shots. A bit embarrassing, really, for the poor jackeroo. He hadn't been employed all that long, couldn't ride too well and was unceremoniously dumped halfway through the shoot.

'What about we head out and you can have a look at how we muster these days? Choppers aren't much good in this area, we really let the cattle muster themselves.'

Everything was just so flat. The ground was a mosaic of pink and cream, yellow and white, a landscape so truly Australian. The artesian bore was a hive of animal activity. Water flowed to the surface through fifteen-centimetre pipes from a considerable depth. It was quite hot and needed time to cool before the cattle could drink. There was a slightly metallic taste although not an unpleasant one. Big Brahmans moved slowly around the long open troughs, slurping water lazily as they wandered here and there searching for their calves. Well over 200 beasts, their massive grey bodies, long floppy ears and pendulous dewlaps swinging in the breeze. Only the odd deep grumbling bellow broke the silence. There was no panic, no excitement, everything they did had a purpose and that was simply to quench their thirst. Water was the magnet and Cath explained how things worked.

'The bore area here is surrounded by a big yard, about twenty acres in all. There are three gates through which the cattle can enter. But once in they cannot get out. It's a self-mustering yard. Saves a lot of time and a lot of manpower.' Andy is recording sound while Rosie takes the shots.

'How do the gates work?' I asked.

'If you look you'll see. As the cattle come in and push their way through the broad end of the funnel the spring-loaded gate will open slightly to allow them to enter, but of course once they're in, the narrow end isn't wide enough to allow them out.' Such a simple idea and yet so practical.

We stepped outside the yard and walked back through the dancing haze to the vehicle.

'I'll need to record an atmos,' called Andy to Rosie. 'Could you all stand still and be quiet for sixty seconds?' He slipped on the cans (earphones to you), Rosie rolled the camera at absolutely nothing and the sounds were recorded.

But there was no sound. It was so quiet that until you stopped and listened very closely you'd never notice the complete tranquillity. A bird flew past some twenty-five metres away. Andy looked up.

'What was that?' Against a background of such total silence, the noise of a bird on the wing was overwhelmingly audible.

The horizon was punctuated with little spirals of dust – each one a beast or two on their way in to get a drink. Watching, it seemed to take hours for the shape of a cow to appear out of these greyish coils of sand and clay, but then, everything moved so slowly here, even time itself.

'They'll walk in from over ten miles to get a drink,' Cath said. This was quite a place. A place that defies description, but this is Australia, the real Australia, and we'd been lucky enough to record it for all to see.

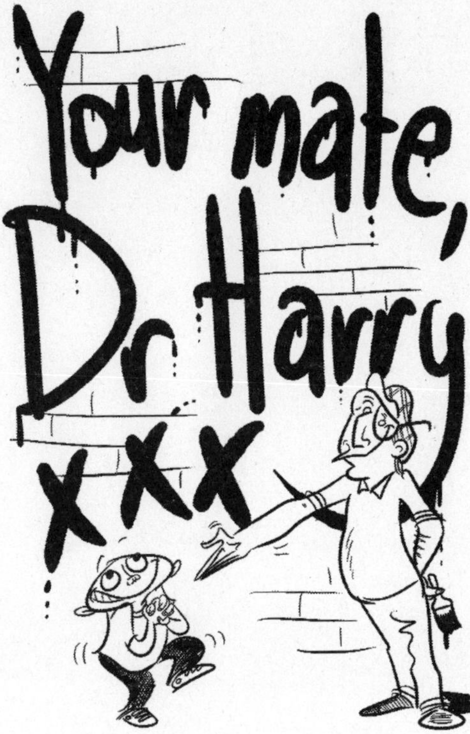

Expos

10

Over Expo-sed

'Talk to the Animals' had been up and going for over twelve months when the first of what was to become a very regular event took place. It was around the end of February, and the venue was to be Sydney's old showground out at Moore Park. The Seven Network was involved, as part of the overall sponsorship, I think, and posters with the now-familiar face of Dr Harry appeared all over billboards and television screens right around the city. The expo was unconnected with 'TTTA' in any way, but had yours truly as its star attraction. Remembering that we used to live in Sydney, the idea of having such an extravaganza at the time of year when the heat and humidity of summer are at their very worst seemed to Janine and me just a little crazy. To have it in what we well remember as the old Sample Bag Pavilion, where any sizeable crowd would virtually choke the place, seemed a little peculiar.

It was out of our hands but we went, with a wombat, Lucille, in tow for good measure. Of the three of us, I think Lucille enjoyed it the most. Channel Seven went out of their way to look after us. Transport everywhere was by luxury Mercedes with leather seats and uniformed chauffeur. Our hairy little Tassie friend took it all in her stride. There have been very few of her kind that have managed to clock up as many frequent flyer points as Lucille has. The rooftop penthouse of the York Apartments sits right at the city end of Sydney

Harbour Bridge, and I have related elsewhere Lucille's fascination with the peak-hour traffic. For the full three days we spent in absolute luxury I'm certain none of the staff realised there was a third party in the room. She had an absolute ball. Racing all over the joint, and ricocheting from one wall to another like some over-charged dodgem car. Janine had brought all the food along. Weet-Bix, cat biscuits, fruit of every description, even her own Tasmanian bottled water – you see, to my wife, aside from her family, animals really are the most important things around.

Come the first morning and we were collected from the foyer at around ten o'clock for the trip to the expo. No one really knew what to expect. This was the first day. Parking spots appeared to be at a premium even outside the grounds, and it took some time for the Merc to navigate its way through the people and vehicles crowding around the entrance. It's a strange feeling to look out a car window and see total strangers waving at you, even calling your name. Everywhere I looked there were massive posters advertising the event and each one featured my bespectacled face and cloth cap. Wow! This thing seemed from the word go to depend on a fella who up until a year or two ago was just a struggling vet. I swallowed hard, smiled and waved – feeling, I must admit, a trifle embarrassed by the whole event. Janine, too, was overawed. Lucille just kept chewing on a carrot.

The driver managed to get us in via the back entrance and the 'Talk to the Animals' crew were there to do a spot of filming before I was supposed to do a bit on stage. Quite frankly we were hard-pressed to get much material. In short, there were very few animals there at all! Two or three quick bits with a camel and a cow, and an amusing aside with a horse that managed to bite me rather hard on the forearm were about it.

My stage appearance was pretty brief. At one corner of the pavilion the organisers had erected a low platform and some hundred or so chairs that they thought would suffice as a mini presentation area. It was hopelessly inadequate. Lucille and I did our bit, talked about wildlife and how important our native animals were, and so on. Fully ten minutes and that was it. Then the three of us were escorted to the Channel Seven stand, a flimsy structure situated somewhere near the middle of the pavilion, to sign some autographs.

This was my first experience with fan cards and with strangers asking me to write various messages to them and sign my name. This is what fame is about, or is it really? Fame is perhaps the most fleeting of all human conditions. In years to come people will say, 'Harry? . . . Harry who?' And that will be that. Enjoy it while you can is the answer, but always remember your roots and be humble.

There was not a big crowd on the Friday, and although the day was a warm one there was enough room to move around and see things – but, quite honestly, there was very little to see. By three o'clock people were leaving and it was time for the three of us to return to our unit as well. Tomorrow is another day.

Saturday was indeed just that. By the time we arrived the mercury had climbed to the mid-thirties. Janine was concerned for Lucille's safety, and had packed a couple of wet towels and freezer bricks to keep her cool; after all, she was a native Tasmanian. The crowd was very much bigger. People were everywhere. Just getting inside with the car proved an effort. The people were different too. Not happy and smiling like the day before. Grim-faced and angry would be more like it.

'Where's the bloody animals?' . . . 'Where do you get a drink?' . . . 'Where's the damn taxis?' This bloke with two kids in tow confronts me. 'There are no animals here!' he exclaims. He was right, there weren't. It took fully ten minutes to get inside the pavilion. I sent Janine on ahead with the wombat, while the driver and I battled through the abusive crowd. Inside and safely behind the stage we sat and recovered our composure. Nothing like this had ever happened before. People were holding me personally responsible for the whole shemozzle. The lack of animal exhibits. And there were very few – thank heavens for Parks and Wildlife and their praying mantises. Unfortunately it turned out to be just a trade show. A maze of dog kennels, fish tanks, feeding bowls and leads. Boring with a capital 'B'. These people had come to see animals. Dr Harry was the face on the poster and it seemed to them that Dr H was personally responsible for the whole damn mess. In retrospect, because the concept of an expo like this was new, it's possible the organisers just underestimated people's love for living creatures, their interest in seeing animals.

The compere welcomed Lucille and me on stage, asked a few amusing questions, we rabbited on about this and that and after ten minutes it was over and time to head off to the Seven stand for more autographs. The booth was about seven metres square and built from lightweight aluminium to make assembly and transportation easy. On two sides there were narrow counters and the remainder was filled in with a small shed where the staff could seek refuge from the throng. Janine and Lucille stood behind me as I perched on a stool behind one of the counters. There was no order to things. The crowd in front was some ten deep. Many were still yelling expletives about the conduct of the event. The whole thing had a bad atmosphere.

Something inside told me this was not going to be a nice experience. I started to sign, smiling all the time and trying to make pleasant conversation and light of the problems.

The crowd pushes ever closer. There is no orderly line, just a mass of fairly dissatisfied people, and Janine's husband is the target of their anger.

Without warning the mob surges forward, the stand lurches ominously, and begins to topple slowly backwards. I'm still trying to remain calm, and keep signing and smiling, in that order. The stool starts to slip over as well. This is dangerous. Now the whole structure is listing badly and I fall from the stool. 'Get him out of there before we're all killed!' yells Janine. And she wasn't kidding. It took a good five minutes before any sort of security arrived to eventually restore order. An angry crowd is something I hope never to encounter again. Everyone thought this was my expo! Every poster had my face smack bang in the middle of it; who could blame them? It was a nasty experience. Even Lucille was visibly upset.

Janine is a lady of few words, but very well-chosen ones. 'We won't be back tomorrow,' she told the organisers, 'unless there's damn good security!' Sunday was indeed a better day. Nowhere near as hot, and some food and drink stands had suddenly materialised. The word had obviously got out as well because there were far fewer people in attendance. It came time for the afternoon stage appearance, and as Lucille and I readied ourselves backstage for what would be our last appearance on the podium I heard Janine whisper, 'Tiffany's out there.'

'What did you say?'

'Tiffany is out there . . . I can see her standing at the back of the crowd.'

'Go and get her. Bring her back here.'

It was time to go on. Most people will tell you that wombats are dumb animals. Don't you ever believe it. Animals sense every emotion we display, yes, even wombats. Neither of us wanted to be out there, but the show must go on. In spite of all the turmoil that was unravelling my nervous system . . . the show must go on. My mum had told me that a thousand times in my youth and now in spite of all the trauma whirling and spinning within my brain, we would do it. When every part of me wanted to be backstage. Back with a lost child, a daughter that we hadn't seen for nearly seven years. My firstborn. Tiffany had come back. She had made the move to heal the scars of time and separation, and we will always love her for it. Thank you, my darling wife, for seeing her in the crowd. I couldn't pick her out but you did. Perhaps it was that you wanted to see her, that's what I've always believed.

What do you say to a child you thought you had lost? You don't say much. You cry a lot, you hug, you squeeze, you let that static charge living within every one of us arc across the river of years and weld two people together again. Ah, just so much to talk about. All those wasted years. Janine is crying too! It's a wonderful time. We sit. We talk. We talk a lot. 'Tomorrow is your birthday,' how could I not remember. Twenty years old. 'We'll celebrate!' declares Janine. 'Our chauffeur will take you home tonight and tomorrow, don't worry.' Worry! That was the farthest thing from anyone's mind. So it was from the mayhem of an animal expo, we salvaged the greatest prize of all. Our daughter. And although Janine is not her mother we don't go for this 'step' and 'half' stuff. She is our child and Heidi's sister.

11

Another Expo Security Blanket

It wasn't too much longer down the track when I was approached to do another of these expos. 'He'll do it for you,' says my lovely wife, 'providing you supply adequate security, and I mean, really adequate'. It was to be in Queensland at the Brisbane exhibition grounds, or the 'Ekka', as the locals call it. The event was sponsored and organised by a totally different company. I was to represent a dog and cat food producer. Janine took over the whole shebang. Overseeing flights and accommodation. There was no way this one was going to end up like the Sydney shambles. You could count on that.

It was business class seats all the way from Launceston via Melbourne. This was already looking very much better than the Sydney one! Seated in the front row we were naturally first off the plane when it touched down in Queensland's capital. No sooner had we stepped from the aircraft than I was accosted by this rather large gentleman. His physique could best be described as an inverted triangle. The guy stood some five centimetres shorter than me but outweighed my puny frame by at least ten kilos. He was all muscle . . . enough said. Dark hair, dark suit, at least three days' growth on a burnt olive face, and fists that could have pulverised any opponent. 'Dr Cooper.'

'Yes,' I hesitatingly replied.

'Good,' he said abruptly, 'follow me.'

'Who is he?' whispered Janine.

'I dunno, but he's bigger than both of us and I'm not arguing.'

As we walked along the narrow corridor leading from the plane to the terminal buildings more of the same people began appearing from the shadows. First another two, one on either side of us. Then two more behind, and lastly a woman on her own bringing up the rear. Bloody hell, there are six of them now. All in charcoal suits, white shirts and narrow, sombre ties. None of them saying anything, as they usher the two of us down a narrow set of stairs. 'This isn't the normal way out!' I protest to the fella in front.

'It is our job, sir, to get you in and out of this airport safely.'

OK, Harry. Best to shut up. Finally at the carousel we stand to one side.

'May I have your luggage checks, sir?' They're handed over with an air of resignation.

'Who are these people?' asks my darling wife.

'I have no idea, but they're getting our luggage.'

'We are your security for the whole weekend,' replies the first guy we met. Obviously overhearing Janine's question.

'Right,' commands another of the group, 'time to go.' And go we did. Straight through the terminal like some human triangle.

All the time Janine is asking, 'Are they all right? Who sent them? Who are they, anyway?' and all other nebulous female questions to which quite frankly I had absolutely no answer. Three black Commodores stood parked at the curb.

'This one, please,' as the doors are opened and the two of us placed like valuable cargo inside the vehicle. Heaven knows where the luggage ended up but we're on our way. At last the driver introduces himself. He's the leader of the team. They are a private security organisation hired for the specific purpose of protecting the two of us from the time we arrived until our departure on Monday morning. The cars travel in convoy. Line astern.

'This must be a movie!' Janine blurted.

'No movie here, madam, this is a training exercise.' A training exercise – and we are the poor devils in the middle of it.

At the hotel, everything is taken care of by the team. We are introduced to the six of them by the boss. Five fellas and one female. And told of the departure schedule for the morning. We are escorted up to our suite in one of my favourite hotels, The Heritage, right on the banks of the Brisbane River. It's to be a 7.30 a.m. breakfast and an 8.15 departure for the Ekka. My darling was in her element. A few days away from young Heidi and the chance to relax in a nice hotel while I did the work. 'Better set the alarm for 6.30, I reckon, you'll be an hour or so getting ready.'

'No, 6.45 will do, I can be ready in that time.' So 6.45 it was.

We had been up and about for some twenty minutes the next morning when there was a loud rapping on our door. To my total surprise, on the other side of the door stood our number one security man. He looked just a trifle ruffled. 'Didn't sleep too well?' I enquired in a rather caring manner.

'Not really, sir.'

'Oh, where did you sleep then?'

'I didn't, sir.'

'Well, what have you been doing all night?' I demanded.

'Standing right outside your door, sir . . . Are you nearly ready for breakfast?'

'Yes . . . give us a minute,' and I slammed the door.

'Who was that?' asked Janine from the depths of the bathroom.

'You're not going to believe this,' I said, 'that big bloke has been standing right outside our door all night. He'd have heard every word.' Janine went scarlet!

A mate had joined the number one guy as we entered the lift and descended to the patio area for breakfast.

'Table for two,' commanded our minder to the scrawny breakfast waiter.

'Shouldn't that be a table for four?' he enquired, having distinguished himself with his mathematical precision.

'I said, a table for two,' repeated our man, who in the eyes of the waiter had suddenly grown several centimetres and twenty kilos. 'This way, please,' and we were shown a lovely table for breakfast.

Our two friends had now joined another two and the four of them were seated in a far corner, drinking black coffee. Keeping one eye on us and one on the time.

The convoy escorted us to the showgrounds and the group took turns all day to keep us under surveillance. This was only a two-day expo and Saturday night we elected to take a stroll around Southbank after dinner. Have you any idea how good it feels being accompanied everywhere you go by a bunch that look like they work out in the gym for twelve hours, seven days a week, in the seediest part of town? You can stop and check out whatever you like without the slightest worry. They were six really nice people and their boss, who was wheelchair-bound, was a top guy too. I remember as kids we would often walk down the street toward a group of other kids. We'd yell 'split' and hope they did or there'd be a blue. This was like the old days. Everywhere we went the human triangle surrounded us and cut through the crowds like a hot knife through butter.

By lunchtime Sunday it had all got too much for that wife of mine. 'I can't stand this any longer,' she said, 'that damn woman follows me everywhere . . . I'm going to give her the slip and have some time to myself.' With that she was gone. The stand was busy, with autographs for me to sign and so many questions to answer. Back then most of the problems related to scratching dogs; these days they are more related to behavioural matters.

It must have been well over two hours before Janine returned. 'I was beginning to worry about you,' I confessed.

'No need to do that,' she retorted. 'That damn woman [who incidentally resembled a Russian female weight-lifter who had OD'd on anabolic steroids], she followed me everywhere!'

'But that's their job,' I protested.

'Too bad. I slipped away from her and ducked behind a couple of stands selling pottery, crawled under two trucks and then crossed down two rows and got tangled with a bloke selling palm trees and a lady with alpacas. Couldn't see her anywhere, so I slowed down and had a good look around. Just when I thought it was time to get back I slipped into the loo. You're not going to believe this,' she went on. I believe anything she tells me. 'There I am seated on the throne. Knickers around my ankles, relaxing and thinking I've done well, when there's a knock on the door.

' "Mrs Cooper . . . Mrs Cooper, it's Security. Are you all right in there?"

'A woman can't even have a pee in private.'

We look back and smile these days at our first big protective experience. Although it may have been over the top, as they escorted us up the gangway and onto the jet for our flight home they still maintained the closest and most professional attendance of any security group with which I've been associated.

12

The Biggest Expo of All

Life's experiences should all teach us something. Some people have twenty years' experience in a field. Other people have the same experience every year for twenty years. We can all benefit from the sharing of such knowledge.

With all that in mind, the producers of 'Talk to the Animals' decided to put together their very own animal extravaganza. It turned out to be the most fantastic animal event that I've been part of. The venue would be perhaps the most important facet of the whole event. Rather than choose an old tired site like a showground, they wisely went for something that was modern, well-known, had plenty of open space and yet provided cover if the weather turned nasty. An occasion like this needs to attract families, and give them a full day's entertainment for their admission fee. Caulfield Racecourse was selected as the preferred site and an inspirational choice it proved to be, for here in the one area was everything needed to make the event a success.

Things like this don't just happen, they take a tremendous amount of planning and knowledge to make them a success. Right from the start a team was employed specifically for the purpose. They set about the task, armed with the knowledge of hindsight from all the problems of the Sydney experience. The date would be late October, not too cold and not too warm, with a fairly good chance of fine weather. It was billed as the 'Talk to the Animals Expo'. With the television series rating its head off, and Melbourne being one of our strongest viewing regions, all of us on the show knew we were in for a memorable time. Where everything had been wrong in Sydney, everything was right in Melbourne.

The publicity for the event was unprecedented: television, radio and print media were used to great advantage. Everyone in Melbourne and the surrounding countryside knew what was going on. The name was on everybody's lips. It was just a matter of fingers crossed for good weather and the people should come.

The expo would run over four days: Thursday to Sunday. All the closed-in area under the grandstand was set aside for various commercial exhibitors. Cat and dog food, accessories of every kind, birdseed and cages packed the floor space. A huge cat show staged over the whole four days attracted record entries and the public was able to witness all the exotic breeds, talk with the exhibitors and witness the judging. Likewise a huge dog show ran in conjunction, though obviously well away from the cats. Every afternoon the winners were paraded on a stage, and the results and merits of this and that breed discussed with an eager audience. So many different breeds on display each day made for an ever-changing focus. The trophies were unique. One-offs to celebrate the expo.

The ferret club was in attendance. Rabbits of every size and breed hopped around at least three displays. The mouse club had a steady stream of young and enthusiastic visitors. Not one but three different alpaca studs vied for attention, then there were the llamas, goats and fancy sheep. Horse and pony rides, and authentic working farriers who spent the whole four days making shoes from scratch and shoeing the many horses on display. Palominos, Clydesdales, Welsh and Australian ponies . . . well over a dozen different breeds. For the bird enthusiasts, poultry clubs had combined to display an enormous range of fancy fowl, ducks and geese. There were pigeons, cockatiels and budgerigars, finches and canaries. If it had feathers it was sure to be there. Cattle, of course, buffalo and deer, all safely ensconced inside strong yards, but many with young at foot tethered just outside, much to the delight of the thousands of children. If it walked or waddled, flew or swam, it was there. Fish, axolotls, reptiles – the list was endless. There was assembled at the one time and in the one place, the best cross-section of the domestic animal kingdom I have ever witnessed.

At so many other events I've attended prior and since, the animals and the public were kept well separated. A fence or barrier was always in the way; people couldn't touch the animals. There was no hugging and stroking. At this expo people and animals really got together. There were no obstructions. Children hugged and kissed the animals, parents stood back with a smile on their faces and a song in their hearts. This experience was like the agricultural shows of old. No sideshow alley here. No wretched sample bags, fairy floss or kewpie dolls on sticks. Just wall-to-wall animals. Everything alive. Everything warm and soft and cuddly, and everything free (well, all except the camel and pony rides)!

Riding demonstrations and horsemanship displays dominated the main arena, just beyond the finishing post of the racetrack, and the crowd viewed the whole scene from the comfort of the huge grandstand. Not just one but three stages kept the crowd entertained and the five of us from 'TTTA' presented a live show twice daily with dog trainers, snake handlers and the like on the main platform. There was always something happening. Catering was first class. No complaints this time about the lack of food or animals. It was saturation level. A return to the days of old when animals were the centre of attention, not the people!

Come Sunday afternoon Janine, Heidi and I had well and truly had it. My voice was reduced to just a whisper, and the right hand felt like soggy spaghetti; even the effort of holding a pen, let alone signing 'just one more autograph', was beyond imagining. Heidi had purchased her two alpaca outfits, and had collected a swag of photographs from spending most of her time with these adorable animals. Janine had, of course, added to our canine family. 'Don't you think she's just gorgeous?'

I didn't have the strength to disagree. 'We'll call her Pepper.'

'Yes, Dad, that's a great name!' added Heidi, and so a Dandi Dinmont terrier joined Rosie and the Cavaliers. Looking something like a dachshund in outline, but with a silver-grey wiry coat and a massive pompom perched right on top of the head, Dandi Dinmonts are quite a sight. Supposedly bred by the gypsies on the English-Scottish border areas, the first dogs were purchased by some nobleman who enquired as to what they were called. The seller had no idea so the nobleman asked his name. 'Why, it's Dandi Dinmont,' he replied. So the name stuck. Well, it's a good story anyway. Pep is still the character she was as a pup and much prefers life on the back verandah to life in the kennels. I suppose with her little short legs it is hard to keep up.

The event was summed up in many ways when a sergeant of police confronted me on Sunday, halfway through a long, last afternoon. 'Y'know,' he said, 'there's a damn sight more people here today than there were last week and they're a whole lot better behaved.' Last week had been the Caulfield

Cup! Just as well we were there after the cup too, for they had to repair the main straight when we left. The camel rides operated up and down this famous strip of grass – trouble was, everywhere the camels had a pee, they killed everything that was green. You see, camel urine is so very concentrated. Being desert dwellers their kidneys have adapted to such a degree that they absorb every spare bit of water from the yellow fluid. The darn stuff is that rugged it would probably kill concrete!

The expo brought animals and people together in the most intimate fashion. It was touch. It was feel. It was real. An event like this is so all-encompassing that it swamps your whole being. When it's finished emptiness takes hold, but in time comes the realisation that you have been a part of something very, very special. An event that will be talked about for years to come. A unique experience that will have many imitators. Something so special that in the future it will serve as the yardstick by which all others will be measured. I doubt we will ever see the likes of it again.

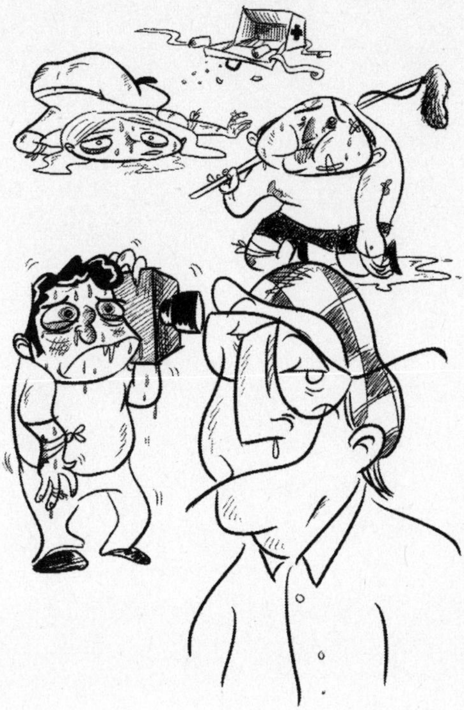

Behind the Scenes

13

Tucker on Tour

There's a perception evident, when I talk to people here and there, that television is a wonderful life.

'Why shouldn't it be?' they ask. 'You fly all over the place, stay in the best hotels, eat the best food, it must be fantastic.'

The answer is, 'yes', there are some really good times when we do exactly that. But these amount to little more than 5 per cent of our time on the road. Travelling is plain hard work. To make a surprise house call, particularly if there is any driving involved, we're up by 6.00, on the road half an hour later and knocking on someone's door by 7.00. Sundays we're a little kinder to ourselves and start half an hour later. To film each story takes a minimum of two and a half to three hours and in some cases a lot longer; the record is seven and a half.

The place was Albury, on the banks of the mighty Murray. They have but one operative paddle-steamer and the guy who runs the boat also owns a Chesapeake Bay retriever whose main problem was that it wouldn't stay out of the water and wouldn't come when it was called. These dogs are born and bred near the water and it's such a natural attraction for the breed that to overcome what breeding has instilled into the animal is difficult to say the least. How to get a dog to come when it's called – that's a bit easier. So we arrived fairly early on a Saturday to catch him before he fired up the boilers for his first trip. We walked the dog up and down the banks, filmed it getting in and out of the water, and then, 'Sorry folks, I've gotta take the boat for a trip.' That's how it was for the whole of the day. We only had him for half an hour or so in between ferry trips. It's more than a little difficult to rivet a dog's attention on you when all it really wants is to ride on the boat. We got there in the end. It was a good dog and using the long lead technique and positive reinforcement with food rewards we were able to get the dog to come to him on command.

Our accommodation had been first class but now we were headed for Yarrawonga, it was late in the afternoon and we had a fair old drive in front of us. My researchers do their very best to give us detailed instructions as to how to get to a place. Finding Yarrawonga was no problem, finding the joint we were staying in, now that's another question. After driving up and down the same road four times and asking two of the locals, each of whom gave different directions, we finally stumbled on the establishment tucked away on the edge of the weir and surrounded by a mass of half-built concrete block units. It was hard to tell whether they were putting them up or pulling them down. The apartments were nice enough, but there was nothing to eat and nothing to drink. Being on the road again at 6.30 the next morning and getting breakfast before then is something of a chore, but the manager on duty managed to sort things out with the local cafe and we left with a decent feed in our bellies. From Yarrawonga, next stop Echuca.

The accommodation was down as a B&B, we don't normally have this sort of thing, motels or apartments are more our go, but this was a wonderful historic house with two delightful hosts who proceeded to shower us with the most magnificent breakfast I've ever encountered. Stunning fruit salads, bacon and eggs with all the trimmings, freshly squeezed juices, all served on antique crockery and in a delightful sunroom overlooking spacious gardens. Yeah, it's nice to be spoilt sometimes, and you feel a bit awkward when your hosts walk in at night and you're eating takeaway pizza on their very collectible lounge. We did enjoy one particularly fantastic meal in town, a restaurant perched right over the river with ancient paddle-steamers below all lit up to provide an atmosphere reminiscent of bygone days. But of all our restaurant experiences over the length and breadth of the country there are a certain few that for one reason or another stand out.

Brisbane's accommodation was usually at the Stamford Plaza, used to be The Heritage, right on the river with magnificent views and equally opulent rooms, breakfast on the river terrace is atmosphere plus, but our favourite restaurant is Pier Nine just down the road no more than ten minutes' walk from the hotel. Over the years we've had some really great times there, but one is particularly memorable.

'I don't think I'll come out with you guys tonight,' says Chris, our intrepid producer. 'I'm a bit tired and I think an early night would do me good.'

'Are you sure?' says Andre the cameraman.

'I'll see how I feel after a shower.'

She felt OK. 'But I don't think I'll drink much.'

We ate everything on the menu. The day had been a wretched one. Nothing had gone right. People weren't home, dogs didn't do what the owners said they would; in fact, absolutely nothing fell into place and we'd arrived back with our tails well and truly between our legs.

'Sod it,' said Andre, 'we're gonna have a good night tonight, things can't get any worse tomorrow.'

'Darn right,' said Steve. And the mood was set for a full-on session. Oysters all round, another couple of interesting entrees to share, mud crabs, Moreton Bay bugs and great slabs of fish punctuated with magnificent chips and fresh green salad, all washed down with copious quantities of Capel Vale something or other. For a girl who wasn't going to have a drink, Chris well and truly did her bit to empty the bottles. We blew all our travelling expenses on one night's meal. Boy, was it worth it!

Next morning it's a seven o'clock start. It's a Sunday. The three blokes are all feeling and looking just a trifle seedy. I'm the last one down for breakfast. Juice and cereal was all I could manage and a cup of very strong tea.

'Hello there, I'm the frog lady from Brisbane.' I feel a touch on my left shoulder and turn to be confronted with the beaming face of an overzealous lady who promptly draws up a chair and proceeds to engage me in avid conversation about all things froglike. At ten past seven most of the cerebral synapses have yet to become activated and the brain is struggling to remember just who this woman is.

'You remember me, of course . . . I'm the frog lady . . . you came to see me . . . I told you all about frogs.' I swear I've never seen her in my life before.

'I can't quite place you,' I replied, stalling for time and hoping that some vague recollection might spring from the vaults of my memory. No such luck. 'Are you sure it was me?'

'Yes, I'm certain.' I was just as certain it wasn't. But she kept babbling on just like the brook beside which most of her amphibians would wish to have resided.

'How long ago was it?' I asked, searching for a clue.

'Three or four years.' Ah, the penny dropped, back in the old 'Talk to the Animals' days.

'It was probably that pretty blonde girl who came to see you, wasn't it?'

'Yes, you're right, it was.' How in God's name she confused me with her I wouldn't know. But when you host a television show everyone thinks it's always you that they've seen, not one of the reporters. This woman was unstoppable. I'm pouring another cup of tea, Steve's poring over the paper, Andre's got up and left five minutes ago, I can see him out of the corner of my eye, he's sitting laughing and wiggling his mobile phone. For heaven's sake, Andre, give me a call, I pray. He just keeps laughing. She hasn't shut up for at least ten minutes, this lady could talk under water with a mouth full of tadpoles, I'm trying to be polite, the head's pounding and it's twenty-five past seven – where's Christine?

'I'm off,' announces Steve, striding down to the foyer to take up a position immediately alongside Andre. Now two of the mongrels are laughing. Finally she stops. 'You'll have to excuse me, my producer seems to be a little late for breakfast and I need to see if she's OK.'

'I'll wait 'til you come back.' Golly, I hope there's a back door we can sneak out of without being seen.

The hotel phone rings for about the tenth time in Chris's room.

'Hello,' snaps a raspy contralto voice. 'Who is it?' Boy has she got 'em this morning.

'Chris, it's Harry, are you OK?'

'Of course I'm OK, what's the problem?'

'Well, you said to meet for breakfast at seven o'clock and that was forty minutes ago.'

'Oh s . . .' something told me this was not going to be a good day, but then again, anything had to be better than the frog lady from Brisbane.

In Lonnie (Launceston to you mainlanders!) it's Fee and me, Stillwater and The Metz that drag us in, but then that's home ground for me and the family's a regular at all of these. Down Hobart way there's a little place called Mit Zitrone a short drive out of the CBD, but worth the effort, no risk – it's FBW's favourite haunt and the twice-cooked eggs are his perennial choice. (FBW is Craig the cameraman – otherwise known as Fat Boy Watkins. I explain in *Remedies & Memories* how he came to get this nickname.) It's a BYO and the local cellar always has plenty of the right stuff on hand. Yep, we do enjoy ourselves sometimes. When it comes to accommodation, there's just a place or two that has been a little different.

Take a little motel in country Victoria. In small towns there's often not a lot to choose from and although the office does their very best to come up with the pick of the crop, it's hard to know when you're not there to check the place out personally. The proprietors were a husband and wife who, quite frankly, should have had a holiday two or three years ago or filed for divorce the day before we arrived. Every time the poor bloke opened his mouth, she howled him down. I'm walking in the door of one room as he holds it open, only to be grabbed on the left arm by the good lady screaming excitedly, 'That's not the doctor's room, this is his room!' All spoken while she physically yanks me across the driveway and virtually hurls me headlong into another abode. 'He needs the spa room.' Yeah, but do I really need a spa right at the end of the damned bed? How in God's name do you walk to the other side of the bed without swimming through the spa? Whoever designed this room must have had a bent slide-rule.

At the end of a long day you frankly don't care, all I'm after is a hot shower, a decent feed and a good comfortable bed away from the noise of passing traffic. The shower recess is so small it's a trifle difficult to get out of the way of the trickling water that emanates from the rusting showerhead long enough to get any sort of lather on your anatomy. Everybody else probably has a spa and then climbs straight into bed, I muse, or perhaps they fall out of bed and straight into the spa. The remainder of the bathroom is equally as small. Dry the face, and grope around for the glasses, then finish the rest of the torso. Good God, there are signs everywhere, they needn't have bothered tiling the walls – there are so many instructions all neatly typewritten on card then laminated and glued to the wall that any sort of ceramic wall decoration would have been totally obscured.

'Guests are requested not to remove makeup with any of the towels placed in the bathroom, please use tissues supplied for such purposes. Penalty for breaching this provision, $25.'

'Nail varnish is not to be applied over the basin and surrounds, any nail varnish found contaminating such areas will be subject to a penalty of $25.'

'Perfumes, nail varnish removers and other toxic chemicals are not to be used within the confines of the bathroom. Such materials may cause damage to the laminated surfaces. Penalty for misuse, $25.'

'Guests are supplied with one bath towel and one hand towel per person. Further towels are available from the office, but require a deposit of $25 per towel.'

What a shame I didn't have some twenty-five dollar notes

and thank heavens I forgot me lipstick and nail varnish. But wait, there's more.

'Guests are requested not to eat, drink, smoke, or cut fingernails or toenails whilst in bed. Should cleaning staff find any evidence of such misdemeanours a penalty of $25 will accrue.'

'The air-conditioning has been precisely set for your comfort, do not interfere with the dials. Should you wish to have the temperature varied, please contact reception, failure to do so will result in a penalty of $25.'

And last but not least.

'Please return your key to reception on departure. Failure to return the key will result in the penalty of $50.' I ask you, who'd ever want to come back!

In the main, staff and management are extremely considerate, they make valiant but often failed attempts to shield us from the general public when all we crave after a hard day's work is just a little bit of peace and quiet.

Towards the end of each year I embark on what in the trade is called a book tour. It's a trip around most of the capital cities promoting the fact that 'Yes, folks, I have written and have had published yet another book.' We have combined these public appearances with 'Harry's Practice' visits – it makes sense to share expenses and certainly utilises my time more efficiently.

Adelaide/Perth was the longest tour of the lot. I'd spent two and a half days in shopping centres and the like and it felt good to be looking forward to a nice meal and a good bottle of something special before I launched into three or four days' filming. The day had been a funny one. The venue was some huge glassed-in conservatory set slap-bang in the middle of some regional plaza. The bookseller had set up a table and display out in front of the shop on the main walkway of the first floor. By the time I got there, the queue stretched back for something like forty metres. Boy, it makes you feel good, but worried all at the same time.

The proprietor is smiling, he thinks it's great. Away I go, signing for all my worth, answering questions, talking to the children and enjoying what I like doing most, meeting people who love their animals. Twenty minutes have passed and the queue is getting longer rather than shorter, it's now around the bend.

'How long've I got here?'

'As long as you like, Harry,' replies my publicist.

'Just go along the line and tell all the people to be patient, I won't leave until I've finished, everyone will get an autograph.' You can hear the sighs of relief.

Ten minutes on and we're going well. When out of nowhere storms this Gestapo-like figure clothed in sombre blue, but sprouting some colourful embroidery on her pocket, which suggests she may have a degree of authority.

'Are you Harry?' The question is obviously addressed to me.

'No . . . I'm Dr Harry to you . . . what seems to be the problem?' I say, getting to my feet so I'm now a good twenty centimetres taller than she is.

'There's a chook in the queue.'

'Is he on his own?' I ask, trying to defuse the situation with a little humour.

'He certainly is not,' she replies in a manner that suggests confrontation is just around the corner. 'We don't allow animals in the plaza.'

I looked at the queue, then at the storeowner and then at the security lady.

'Well,' I said, 'look at the situation from this point of view. I realise that animals are banned from most locations such as this but then again, you are on your own here, aren't you?' She nodded. 'I'd say there's the best part of seventy or eighty people back there, wouldn't you?' She looked to the right and grudgingly agreed. 'Why don't we ask everyone if the lady with the chook could come up to the head of the queue and I could look at the chook and provide whatever treatment is necessary and then send her and the chook on their way?'

The crowd grew restless, the storeowner fidgety. When you're confronted with a savage dog, always adopt a position of submissiveness but when the dog is twenty centimetres shorter than you, stare it out – you're gonna win this one, Dr H.

And so it was that I got to examine a glorious crossbred Old English game cockerel with a very severe upper respiratory tract infection. Then having prescribed the appropriate medication and sent my smiling client, her coughing rooster and the grimacing plaza security woman on their way, we were able to get on with the day. But yes, folks, as always, there's more. Just when I thought I'd got to the end of the queue up bowled a lady with a shopping trolley.

'Dr Harry,' she whispered ever so quietly, 'would you mind having a look in here?' She pulled back a thin blanket which covered a small box on the bottom of the trolley to reveal the baldest guinea pig I've ever seen.

Three of us were eating, we'd had a snifter at the bar beforehand and were halfway through our entrees when from behind us the wine waiter attempted the impossible. There is only room for so many glasses on a tray and when one attempts to override that rule pandemonium ensues. Having piled his platter to the brim with empty wineglasses he bent down to add just one more empty to the throng. Bingo . . . the domino effect . . . glasses and glass went everywhere, mainly all over us.

'Sit still, Kate, don't move . . . we're covered in glass.'

Waiters are running from everywhere, they're apologising and removing slivers of glass all at the one time. There are at least three bits on the top of my right hand alone, half a dozen or so on my cap, and perhaps one has gone down the back of my neck.

'Would you like another table, sir, madam?'

'No, just clean this one up, please.'

'Of course we'll bring more entrees.' Everything was covered in glass.

'I'm gonna have to go to the bathroom and get undressed, will you guys be right 'til I get back?' Kate the producer and my soundo nod in acquiescence. Luckily we've all escaped unscathed. The new entrees have arrived and I find the wine waiter carefully decanting yet another bottle of Mr Henschke's very best.

'Where did that come from?' I asked.

'Oh,' said Kate, 'I thought we should have another bottle at their expense, there could have been glass in our glasses [they were damned near empty anyhow and so was the first bottle] and they agreed.' Go, girl . . . Boy, what a night we had!

14

The Frankfurt's Revenge

There's absolutely no doubt about it, Liawenee is the coldest joint in Tasmania. In fact, it's probably the coldest joint in the whole of Australia and here we are, the intrepid crew: FBW on camera, Craig our producer, Steve the soundo and myself heading up to check out a little dog that just refuses to grow any hair. Believe you me, hair is one of the things you're most likely to need in a Liawenee winter. When we film in Tassie the boys usually stay in Launceston and we meet and travel out together in one vehicle, usually a Tarago or a Falcon wagon. You need something with a pretty big rear end to store all the equipment. Particularly the lights, reflectors and kilometres of electric cord that's strung together to make an on-the-spot film set – it's a bit like the boy scouts, you need to be prepared.

It's an early morning start around 7.30, very little time for breakfast, but on the farm you get used to getting up before the sun and I can't function without a belly full of food to start the day. Not so the crew.

'Do we have to go through Deloraine?' asked FBW.

'Sure, mate,' I replied.

'Do you think anything will be open?'

'Sure, they get up early around here.' These days the main road west bypasses the neat little town of Deloraine, but to get to our destination we had to drive through the outskirts.

'Could we stop for just a minute?' FBW was hungry, FB

was always hungry and the rest of the crew thought they could do with a traveller anyhow, as we still had a good hour or so's climb up the mountains to our destination.

There are quite a few takeaway joints up and down the main street.

'This'll do, Harry, this'll do, pull over, Steve.'

It was usually Steve who did the driving. We tumbled out onto the pavement and FBW made straight for the shop. There wasn't too much on the counter that I fancied. The sambos looked OK, but the hot stuff had the sort of appearance that suggested it'd been there for some substantial period of time. I declined the tucker and went for a drink, Steve and the producer did much the same. Not FBW, he's right into it, a couple of sausage rolls and a frankfurt.

There was something about this frankfurt that I thought suspicious right from the word go. Most frankfurts have that deliciously bright red shiny taut skin, full-of-goodness appearance. Not this example, folks, it was pale, skinny and obviously in need of a transfusion. Every bit of sustenance that had once been packed inside its lacklustre casing had seeped into the tepid water in which it was now drowning.

'I'll take that one,' FBW says – an obvious remark, seeing it was the only one still capable of floating somewhere near the surface. The smiling shop assistant retrieved the soggy mess from the water, which now looked redder than the frankfurt, and laid the corpse to rest in what at least appeared to be a fresh roll.

'Sauce, sir?'

'Absolutely.' And FBW smothered the whole frankfurt in copious quantities of tomato ketchup.

It's a pretty trip winding up into the high country in

Tasmania, the forests of myrtle and beech dripping with the early morning dew and the silver shrouds of tattered parachutes hanging from trees as spiders take their rest from their nightly vigil. You can't go fast, it's narrow, twisting and turning bitumen, but then who'd want to when there is just so much to see on the way. You know, that's the thing about Tassie and probably why I love the place so much, there is just so much to see. Mainlanders look at the map – cripes, the place looks tiny – 'We'll rip around there in four or five days.' That's the way they do it in Targa (our annual road race – just ask Jimmy Richards) but it's not the way to really appreciate how much this island has to offer. Take a fortnight, better still, take three weeks. Stop. Stop often, get out, have a look around. So much of what there is to see is not even listed in the guidebooks, you speed past and you miss it and there are just so many hidden treasures that even in our fifteen years down here I doubt we've encountered more than half.

'Geez, it's xyz freezing,' chatters Steve as he steps out of the Tarago – and it sure was. Down around 3 or 4 degrees, I reckon, and it was already after nine. We were here to visit a mini foxie that belonged to a delightful lady whose job it was to run the local meteorological station. Inside her stone home the fire was blazing and everything was warm and cosy. I looked at the hairless dog, we took some history, made a provisional diagnosis, supplied some medication and filmed the lot. We even gave the dog a beautiful lambswool coat to keep him warm over the upcoming winter months.

There was time for a tour of the back garden. Nothing growing here, just a whole lot of instruments set up on various stands measuring everything from temperature to precipitation, wind velocity to humidity. The good lady read all the gauges twice a day, recorded everything with the utmost accuracy and passed the information on to the central weather bureaus. It's a pretty desolate landscape, nothing but exposed rocks covered with cushions of browning green moss and grey tentacle-like fungii. What trees there are struggle to reach any sort of height in the gale-force winds that howl across the high country. Sure, it's inhospitable, but in another sort of way, it's quite magnificent as Mother Nature vents her fury on what was once a proud and verdant landscape.

We said our farewells at the front door and turned our vehicle back down the drive.

'Any of you guys like to have a look at the trout establishment up here?' I asked.

'What do they do?' questioned Steve.

'It's where they milk the trout to produce their yearly crop of fingerlings; fascinating, really.'

'How long will it take us to get back to town?' interjected FBW as we rolled out of the property and onto the main road.

''Bout an hour I reckon, why?' I replied.

'Oh nothing,' said FBW.

The first half of the trip home was fairly uneventful, Steve at the wheel, FBW in the passenger seat, Craig the producer and myself in the back. As usual, we're discussing anything at all except what we're doing. Funnily enough FBW was taking very little part in any of the discussion. Around halfway down the mountain, I noticed something of a change in the complexion and general wellbeing of our cameraman. Being a veterinary surgeon, one learns to read signs. Let's face it, animals can't talk, you have to watch and observe what they do, if you are to reach a diagnosis. FBW was giving some really weird signs.

'How much longer to go?' His tone was now a little more anxious.

'Around twenty minutes, I reckon . . . you OK?' I asked, somewhat concerned.

'Sure, sure, I'm fine . . . just want to know how long it is, that's all.'

'Don't get snappy, FB,' says Steve.

'I'm not snappy,' snaps FB. Dr Harry to the fore. By now I'm firmly convinced that we're looking at a cameraman with a severe case of hyperperistalsis – yes, folks, his guts were on the move. What had begun as a slow walk had increased to a trot and now was about to progress from a canter to a full-blown gallop, you could even hear 'em, all of us could hear 'em.

'Should I pull up, mate?' says Steve.

'No, just keep going,' groans FB, 'how much further?'

'About five minutes less than it was last time you asked,' says Steve in a totally unsympathetic tone.

It's funny how people's facial expressions change with the onset of many forms of illness. FB's face had faded to a somewhat light grey colour, his cheeks were bulging, his eyes watering, his respiratory rate well above normal and his constant question of 'How much further?' was punctuated by multitudinous swallowing.

'Boy, was that you, FB?' called my producer from the back seat. It's freezing outside, but every window in the car is now right down. The odour emanating from the front of the vehicle suggested that something had died about a week ago and those employed in cleaning the vehicle had left it there to compost under the passenger seat.

'Geez, FB, we'll all be dead,' exclaimed Steve.

'Mate, why don't we just pull up and you can get out.

There's a stack of old papers here in the back of the car and we'll just wait. It's still another ten minutes to town,' I suggested.

'No, I'll be right.' One hundred per cent for stoicism; zero for commonsense.

'We'll be there in five minutes, mate, can you hang on?'

'Yeah, Harry, I'll be sweet . . . where are the toilets?'

'Don't worry, son, we'll pull up right alongside.'

'No, we won't,' says Steve, 'I want a decent air space between us and him.'

'There they are, turn right here, Steve, pull up in that car park.'

In a shot FB is out of the car and running. Perhaps that's not quite the right word to describe his rapid but tortured passage from the front door of the Tarago to the only door of the men's loo. How does a man run when his abdomen is about to explode? It's a sort of a hunched-over quick shuffle, making absolutely sure that you put as little stress as possible on the lower part of your enteric anatomy.

Well, folks, he made it. There must have been something really interesting in that toilet block, for that's where FB spent the next twenty-five minutes. He emerged looking somewhat less swollen, certainly less buoyant, but at least the boy was alive and hopefully on the way back to good health.

You'd think he'd have learnt his lesson. Regrettably such is not the case. I've given up walking into takeaways with FBW. He never fails to emerge without some greasy paper bag full of the most unhealthy gastronomic object that fast-food companies can manufacture. But I've never seen him that crook since and he's assured me he never wants to be that bad again. At least frankfurts seem to be off the menu these days.

15

Producers

The standard joke in the industry – and I've probably told it before – is simply this. How do you know if you're talking to a producer at a party? The answer is, don't worry, they'll tell you.

We have three levels of producers. The field producer goes out on location with the camera crew and myself and is responsible for structuring the story. They make sure all the right shots are taken, information is conveyed and that the mood of the whole shoot conveys the right sort of impression depending on the subject with which we are dealing. (Speaking simplistically we shoot about one hour on location for every one minute on the television screen.) Field producers are also responsible for compiling and writing the story when they finally get back to the office. They are also responsible for dealing with problems that may occur along the way, for having all the props that I consider necessary and whatever else may happen to take the crew's fancy along the journey.

They report to the series producer, who schedules the various stories for the upcoming series. They modify and where necessary edit the stories to an appropriate format that fits each particular episode. This also brings with it responsibility for scheduling trips, surgery shoots and the like. On the very top of the pile sits the executive producer, who oversees the whole show on a weekly basis, passing or modifying stories as necessary, before passing the show to go to air.

Naturally enough it's the field producer with whom I spend most time. Each one has their very own God-given talents which they apply to every story we attempt to film.

Debbie's a country girl, she loves nothing more than getting out and about in the back blocks of Australia where the real people live, because it's here that she can utilise one of her many talents. Somewhere along the line Debbie's father had taught her an interesting little trick for summoning cattle from wherever they might be in a paddock. It's almost impossible to imitate this particular sound. To say that it's a 'wah . . .wah . . . wah' wouldn't be quite correct. It's a sort of cross between a Cherokee Indian war chant, the last gasp of a dying dingo and the quack of an appleyard duck. It's made by cupping both hands over the mouth, closing off the nostrils with the first and second finger to increase the nasal tone and then opening and closing the palms to emit the staccato-like symphony that masquerades as a cow call.

There we are, folks, on the side of the Newell Highway not too far out of Dubbo, when Andre the cameraman spies a whole heap of young steers grazing in a paddock. Before anyone has time to issue a note of caution, tripods and cameras are cascading out of the back of the vehicle. The cattle take one look at this heap of equipment, rapidly decide they don't want to be on television and disappear into a dust cloud and the distance.

'Don't worry,' says Deb, 'I can see another mob just a bit further up the road. Let me get out first and I'll call them all over for you.'

The van creeps slowly down the highway till we're level with a mob of about fifty or sixty Angus and Hereford steers.

'Leave this to me,' I love a woman with authority. Deb is out of the car with all the stealth she can muster, slinks slowly towards the mob clustered around a water trough. They look up nonchalantly and go on drinking. She beckons to the car and whispers, 'Get the gear out.'

Now this mob obviously don't mind having their picture taken, their attention is riveted on Deb, every steer in the mob is eyeballing her, a few even come over for a closer look. 'Get set up, boys, and when you're ready I'll get them all over.'

Three minutes down the track, everybody's in 'go' mood. I'm where I should be, we're ready to roll.

'Call 'em now,' whispers Andre. And without any need for further encouragement, Debbie drops to the ground to be out of shot and goes into her cow-call routine. Over the years I've seen cows move, but none moved like this mob, they left the scene like a Saturn Five rocket leaving a launch pad, kicking and mooing and bucking for all they were worth. In less than twenty seconds there wasn't one within a kilometre of the place.

A very dusty field producer staggered to her feet. 'Can't understand it,' she said, 'it always worked back on the farm. They must be different cattle.'

'Just what sort of a farm did you have, Deb?' I managed to ask through the choking dust.

'Oh, it was a dairy farm, we milked cows.'

'Oh well,' I said, 'they were all ladies, weren't they? These guys were the opposite sex, maybe you'd better drop the whole concerto just an octave or two, that way it'll appeal more to the blokes!' You know, I'm sure she went back home and practised it all over again . . . look out, the next mob of cows we run into.

It's hard on the road when you get sick but if you're made of the right stuff you just keep going. Annie was.

Coolangatta and Surfers Paradise were to be our home for the next few days while we compiled our quota of two stories per day of both normal and surprise house calls. Halfway through our sojourn Annie was struck with the most horrible bout of influenza imaginable, you know the stuff I mean: aching all over, thumping headache, runny nose, and complete and absolute lethargy. As the pseudo medico of the party, yours truly was looked upon to dispense all manner of medication to the sick and ailing, humans as well as animals, but Annie was a health nut. She'd fight this thing to the bitter end with healthy foods, vitamins and herbal supplements, even if it killed her. As the days dragged on she got steadily worse, it was hard to say quite honestly whether her symptoms were now due to a combined massive dose of vitamin C and Echinacea or simply the dreaded onslaught of the virus. By the afternoon of the last day she'd had it.

My client lived in the beautiful hinterland above the bustling metropolis of the Gold Coast, so near and yet so far from the frenzied activities of the holiday-makers intent simply on having a damned good time. Up here it was peaceful and serene . . . until the phone rang. That's when all hell broke loose. The problem animal was the family dog, which insisted on attacking anyone and everyone who answered the darned telephone. What a doozey this was!

Annie had reached the end of her resistance and collapsed like a blancmange on my client's lounge where, in between moans and groans, she managed to direct and produce the story. Intermittently raising her head from this supine position she would deliver a line or two of instructions before collapsing back into a state of semi-stupor.

Half the stuff we did outside. The usual bits, like the walk-up. The knock on the door, the 'G'day, how are ya, what seems to be the problem?', 'Let's take a look around', 'Show me the dog', 'Tell me what happens', and then it's time for the demonstration. So I ring on the mobile phone and the moment their fixed-line phone starts to ring, this crossbred Border Collie goes totally ballistic. Round and round in circles, jumping up and down, barking and carrying on and finally biting the poor woman of the house as she picks up the phone to answer my call, what a rotten dog!

'What've you done to try and solve the problem?'

'We get everyone to ring on our mobiles, he doesn't seem worried by them.'

Any sort of working dog is a smart animal and if they're smart, they can be trained. What this dog needed was just a little basic obedience training. It's this simple: the dog would rather eat the treats in my hand than worry about the telephone, so that's just what we taught my client to do. Simply hold the dog in a 'sit' position using food rewards while she calmly picked up the phone and chatted on for as long as she wished. Story done.

It was now nearing four in the afternoon and the possibility of catching an earlier flight home lifted the spirits of the whole crew. Calls were made, bookings changed and, yes, the three of them could fly out that night instead of waiting till the next morning. (Yours truly, living just south of the big river they call Bass Strait, had to wait it out until the next day. Not too many planes fly into Tassie and that was before Ansett imploded.) All the gear was packed and the back door slammed shut on the Tarago. All aboard. Hang on, aren't we missing somebody? Poor Annie had finally flaked, she'd given it her best shot and now lay in a semi-comatose condition on the lounge. Half-dragging, half-carrying her lifeless form out the front door, we got her as far as the verandah. The poor girl really did look like death warmed up.

For the last two days I'd been trying to pour various medications down her gullet, all of which she'd stubbornly refused on the grounds of, 'But Harry, what about the side effects?' By now her resistance both to the virus and to the repetitious pleadings of the entire crew were at their lowest.

Andre, too, had a dose he could feel coming on. 'Why don't you just take a couple of my cold tablets?' he implored the hapless female form now draped over a chair on the front verandah. She bowed her head in acquiescence.

'Is the water safe to drink?' she stubbornly asked the only other female around the place.

'Yes, it's tank water.' Thank God for that, I thought, there's no way her system was gonna handle an attack by any other pathogenic bug about the place.

'Take two,' advised Andre, tearing open the foil pack. With an effort and a few gulps of water the tablets slid painfully down the back of her throat, and she sank back into the chair.

'We'll have to get a wriggle on to catch this flight,' interrupted Andre and summoning what little strength remained, Annie made it up and into the back seat of the Tarago. (At this stage, folks, I too was quaffing megadoses of any drug in the book, be it herbal or otherwise, that might prevent the same organism taking hold of my body. Heaven knows I'd been cooped up in the back seat next to this walking, talking germ factory of a producer for the last ninety-six hours.)

For the conclusion of this story I have to rely on Andre, and it goes something like this. By the time they'd dropped me off back at the hotel and reached the local airport, Andre's medication was starting to kick in and our otherwise limp rag of a producer was being miraculously transformed into a walking, talking human being again.

'Andre, I feel so much better now, those tablets are wonderful, do you think I could just have one little v & t (vodka and tonic)?'

The great thing about the Qantas Club is it gives you a little privacy and a place to unwind before you jet off again to some other destination, but to Annie the best thing about it was the grog was free!

'Do you think another little v & t would hurt, Andre?'

'Just go a bit easy,' he said. 'Those tablets I gave you don't always mix too well with the grog.'

'Oh, just one more, I can't even taste the vodka.'

By the time the crew boarded the plane Annie had already taken on board three 'little v & t's' and, boy, was she feeling good. So good that she had another two on the plane between Surfers and Sydney. She didn't need an aeroplane, this girl was flying!

'Where are the tapes?' Andre asked as Annie hurried to catch up.

'You've got them, haven't you?' the stunned producer replied.

'No way, I've got the camera, *you've* got the tapes.'

'But I haven't, Andre, *I haven't*!'

The safekeeping of the field tapes with their hours of work, pictures and dialogue, has always been and will always be the sole responsibility of the field producer.

'Where the hell are they?' Andre's frustration was beginning to show.

'Hell, I must have left them on the plane.' The fog cleared, but the flow of passengers leaving the aircraft did not.

'You've got to let me back on, you've just got to, I've left a very important parcel in the locker above my seat.'

'And just what seat was that, madam?' queried the somewhat officious uniformed security man at the top of the aisle.

'Oh God, I don't remember.'

'Do you have a boarding pass, madam?'

Yes, thank heavens she did have one of those buried somewhere in the bottom of her handbag, which could have doubled as a small briefcase. The somewhat tattered cardboard relic was retrieved and so was the parcel of tapes. But wait, folks, there's more.

Wonderful, patient Andre stood waiting for her return. I suppose he felt a bit responsible for the whole episode, having administered the flu medication in the first place.

'Oh, Andre, I've just gotta slip into the loo for a minute, I'll see you downstairs at the baggage carousel.'

'OK,' retorted Andre as he hurried off to collect his vehicle from the valet parking lot.

Twenty minutes have elapsed, everyone on the flight is grumbling, no sign of the luggage. Then the lights flash, the buzzer sounds and the conveyor belt swings into action. Andre and the soundo are busy loading their gear onto those stupid directionless trolleys that cost an even more ridiculous three dollars to rent.

'Where are the tapes?' asked Andre.

'I left them with you when I went to the loo.'

'Oh no you didn't!' Andre was short, sharp and measured in his response.

'Heavens, I've left them in the toilet!'

The scene at the upstairs ladies toilets was like something

out of *Terminator 2*. The door was barricaded and two large uniformed security guards stood in front legs astride, their arms folded in menacing defiance.

'You can't go in, lady.'

'But I need to go to the loo, it's urgent,' blurted Annie.

'There's another toilet just down the corridor, Miss.'

'But I need to go to this one.'

'I'm sorry, madam, but there's a suspect package in one of the cubicles and the bomb squad and sniffer dogs are currently checking the place out.'

'But it's my package, they're my tapes.' she pleaded.

'*Your* package, madam?' Now they were really interested.

The tapes were finally retrieved and this time placed safely in Andre's hands. Annie went home and collapsed; we didn't see her at work for another three days. It's hard to say whether this absence was due entirely to the flu or perhaps a few too many 'little v & t's'.

16

Scary Stairs and Menacing Magpies

There is a saying in television: 'What happens on the road stays on the road.' In other words, the things that go on when you're on a trip away, travelling round the country remain a secret that is to be shared by only those in the know. Well, too bad! Some of these stories are just about to see the light of day.

When 'Harry's Practice' sets out on an expedition to gather both surprise and what we'll call 'ordinary' house calls, the team consists of a producer, either male or female, a cameraman, a sound recordist and of course Dr H, complete with the trusty old black bag. There is always a heap of luggage and there's often consternation at airport check-ins where anywhere between fifteen and twenty pieces of luggage are wheeled up to the counter. Some of this stuff is pretty bulky. The camera legs, the lighting equipment, all the accessory stands, reflectors and the like take up the whole rear end of a Tarago and more than fill three of the meagre airport trolleys. Then there's our own clothing and the props. We have to carry not only a miniature veterinary clinic for any medical problem that might be encountered, but these days a million and one toys, treats, playthings, and amusements to pacify and occupy the animal behaviour problems that seem to be commonplace these days.

As a general rule on these trips we go prepared for just about anything, because when you arrive at the location absolutely anything can happen. The producers really love animal behaviour problems, often because I can demonstrate an immediate solution. For the first three years of 'Harry's Practice' I was to work very closely with the only male field producer on the show. A guy that we all now know as 'Dr Evil' – not for anything that he had actually done on television, but rather for what he has done after hours. Anyhow, that little bit will remain a secret. He was a super producer. A man with the Cecil B. De Mille approach to everything. Well before the departure date he would spend hours on the phone planning and determining every possible scenario that we might stumble upon at each and every venue. Nothing was left to chance. Hence the other nickname of 'CB'.

By now you're wondering just how this whole process comes about. Wonder no longer. We advertise in the local paper of the region, say Kiama on the south coast of New South Wales, that 'Harry's Practice' will be visiting the vicinity in the near future and if you have any animal problems we would love to hear from you by letter, fax or email. These ads can produce up to 800 replies. It's then up to the team of researchers in the office to sort out what they think are the top thirty or forty. They come down to me in Tassie. We have a phone hook-up and pick out the best with a few backups. Then CB gets on the blower and between us we try to create both entertaining and informative television. Sometimes it works. Seldom is everything just as the letter suggests. Often it's the reverse and we're flying by the seat of our pants. ' I'll just have to wing it, mate' is the frequent phrase, and you do the best you can with what's available.

Launceston is my home town and it's not often that we actually film house calls in the region, mainly because people can visit the local surgery at Mowbray and have a consultation there. Exceptions often make the rules. The venue was a kitchen factory; you know, the type of place where they plan, design and assemble that dream kitchen. It was a big factory with around a dozen employees, cutting and sanding for some ten hours a day. The owner of the complex had his office well above the factory floor. It sat right over the top of the building's entrance foyer, and was at least one and a half floors above ground level. No doubt he could keep a keen eye on the goings-on below from his perch on high, but there was one big snag. The only way up was via a spiral steel staircase, and his faithful springer spaniel had for the last three and a half years refused to climb the stairs. She would sit patiently at the bottom, emitting a fearful howl till he walked back down, scooped her up and carried her up all one and a half turns of the stairs. She was no lightweight. Springers are a lot bigger than cockers.

This was no surprise, the owner knew we were coming. CB and the rest of us checked out the location, the dog, and the possibilities of a solution. Half an hour spent on the phone a few days before had shed no light on how to tackle this one. 'Geez, mate,' I exclaimed, 'who'd have thought the stairs would look like this?' The letter had suggested something very different and the props that'd been shipped from the office weren't going to do any good here.

The golden rule of every story on behaviour problems says the animal must display the problem. It's no good just talking about it. It has to happen.

'OK, can you go up to your office and give the dog a call?' I encouraged our bemused dog owner, and obediently he shot up to the landing outside the office door and called to the dog. She was obviously terrified by those stairs. Approaching with a mixture of fear and caution she would put only one paw on the bottom rung, then back off, sit down and start to whimper. Three times we tried it and three times the dog refused to budge; in fact, each time was worse than the last. 'Right,' says CB with the authority that only he could muster, 'now we can all see the problem, Harry. Go ahead and fix it.' (He would add on the odd occasion 'and by the way, we've only got twenty minutes, because there's another one to go to.' The fact that some of these 'problems' had been unsolved for years never seemed to cross his mind. He was on a mission and even I had to fit in with his schedule.)

Dogs, and in fact many other animals, can be frightened by certain objects, particularly if they have never experienced them in their early lives. That's why puppy preschools and early dog training and obedience classes are so important. If puppies learn to cope with 'new things' and conquer that fear at an early age then you seldom have problems later on. Many dogs will not walk over grates in the gutter or over older style wooden bridges, and many dogs will not climb stairs like these. The design was very basic. Simple flat steel treads, with an open balustrade round the outside. This dog felt that once standing on a stair she was 'suspended in midair' because she could see open spaces between each step and through the open balustrade as well. This was a real fear and the object was to help the dog conquer that fear.

'Listen, CB, this is not as easy as it looks, the dog needs to feel secure when it's climbing those stairs.'

'Even I can see that,' was the rather terse reply, 'so just how are you going to fix it?'

'We need to cover in all the gaps between those step treads and cover in the balustrade as well. The dog must think it's in some circular sort of tube, so it can't see the floor below or out into space.'

CB was inventive, I have to give him that. In no time he and the crew had assembled the greatest assortment of carpet off-cuts, packaging material, foam and cardboard, and taped them all over the offending structure. In the meantime I had the springer with me. Teaching some basic obedience, using food rewards to get the dog's attention and to give her confidence in me and my commands. I should perhaps mention at this juncture that the constant carrying of pocketfuls of Supercoat treats in my pockets causes a certain amount of chagrin to my wife when the damn stuff ends up in the washing machine with all my other apparel.

The structure was complete and the time to test it was at hand.

'Andre, you're only going to get one shot at this. I'm going to send the owner halfway up the stairs. I'll lay a treat or two on about the fourth or fifth step so she'll have to get all four feet off the ground to get to them and I'll be up on this big box leaning over the rail to talk to her.'

CB muttered his final instructions. The owner was in place. I led our patient over to the bottom of the stairs. 'Sit,' she sat on command. 'Stay,' she did exactly as I said. This was a good dog, a real good dog. Climbing up on the box I called 'Come,' she put both feet on the bottom step and halted. Looked around at the bits of this and that dangling over what had been for three and a half years an object of terror. 'Come.' All four feet were on the steps. She took the first food reward. Another step. She took the second. 'Call her, call her now,' and the owner did but she panicked, turned around and went back down. She had climbed up six steps.

'She's never ever been up that far in her life!'

'Well, that's great!' Even CB was happy.

'I'll need another shot,' drawled Andre.

'Come on, mate . . . give the dog a go.' I was frankly annoyed, and very much on the dog's side. 'OK, OK, but you'll need to give me another half hour with the dog.' In the back alley behind the factory that springer and I worked like a machine. She was so focused that I felt, well, just perhaps, she might do it again. It was my turn to give the orders.

'Listen CB, this is definitely it. I want the owner to go about halfway up the stairs, here are a few treats for him to give on the way, and he must say 'come', not her name, all right?' I was still a bit annoyed about the whole thing – these sorts of instant solutions don't always come off. Fix a problem that had been around for that long, in less than two hours? Impossibilities we do all the time. Miracles take a little longer.

Over we walk again. The workers on the factory floor are taking bets. Not one reckons she'll go up again. 'Sit . . . Stay,' I'm in position. So is the dog's owner. 'Once she starts climbing you keep calling and move up those stairs on your bum till you get to the landing . . . OK,' Andre's rolling. 'Come,' and she does, straight up this time taking one, two, three treats on the way. She gets to my hand pushed through a hole in some cardboard, takes the treat, goes to turn back. 'Call her. Call her now!' He does, she sees him and responds. Without a glance to the side or above she races up the last ten steps and almost bowls him over with excitement at the top. I'm crying. CB is delighted. The owner holds the dog in his arms. The boys below can't believe it. After all this time she's done it.

'Well done, Dr Harry,' confides CB, 'well done.'

'Not me, CB,' I reply, 'just a real good dog. All I did was help her to conquer fear. She did it, no one could do it for her. It was up to her.' And, you know, I'll always admire her for it.

Then comes the end of the story. The bit where I have to summarise what's happened and talk about the future. So I start describing the structure as 'a packet of poo tickets' – an expression often used by my dad to conjure up the image of a total abomination. 'You can't say poo tickets on television,' pipes up CB.

'Why not?'

'You just can't, that's all.'

'OK, what about "wigwam for a goose's bridle"?'

'Where do you get all this crazy stuff?' CB asks again.

'Just things my parents used to say.'

'All right, say it!'

I did. They cut it out in the edited story, but I managed to slip it in right at the very last. So there you go, a wigwam for a goose's bridle rides again. All the stuff we had used to disguise the staircase was gradually removed over the next few weeks and now the dog races up and down the stairs like they aren't even there.

The CB expeditions have included a visit to our northern neighbours in the Sunshine State. Once again the subject was stairs. This poor geriatric Labrador refused to climb the back stairs of a typical broad verandahed period Queensland homestead to say g'day to his old master. The owner couldn't come down to meet the dog, since he was badly crippled by a severe infection, following a stint in hospital for a relatively minor bone operation. A point not lost on our sound recordist for the day, who was about to undergo a very similar piece of surgery in the near future. There wasn't much else to the story.

Something had given this dog a terrible fright way back when, and ever since the poor old fella just wouldn't go near them. No one really knew why.

'Only one way to fix this, CB, we'll need to disguise the stairs.' The words had no sooner left my mouth than the skies grew black and ominous, someone up there turned on the cold tap and it bucketed down. Everything except the precious camera was wet.

'What do we need, Harry?'

'Probably have to build a ramp and then cover it and the rails with blankets.' Sounds easy, doesn't it, but try to find all this stuff in a backyard that is rapidly disappearing underwater. In spite of it all, timber was found in an old stack, but the incline was too steep.

'Need to make it less of a climb,' I advised, 'this is no frisky pup.'

So precariously perched on broken bricks and rubble that masqueraded as concrete, the bridge over the now very troublesome waters was constructed. Blankets salvaged from the throw-out bag were scattered over everything so the whole apparatus began to resemble a rummage sale at the local hippie commune. No doubt about it, though, up went the dog, just as soon as the old fella called him. Not for my usual food rewards but for, of all things, a big feed of carrots. Congratulations all round; we'd solved yet another one, and we celebrated with a protracted lunch. Filming in the rain was just far too hard . . . well, that's what we told the office.

It was only a day or so later that the intrepid foursome was at it again, this time with a very different story. Something right out of left field. A young fella up in Brissie had been so badly attacked by a magpie last breeding season that he'd all but lost an eye. It was up to us to put together a piece on how to prevent magpie attacks. First you have to recreate the scene. Off to the park we go, complete with this brave young lad and his dad who warns me that, 'This is the park up ahead, and as soon as we step onto the grass I reckon he'll attack.'

Like a replica of General Patton, CB is poised, binoculars pressed hard in to each optic socket. He scans the trees at the far end of the park. 'I see him,' the orders are given with military precision. First to the cameraman, 'Get those heads up and start rolling straight away, it could happen any second,' then to the soundo, 'Keep that damn big fluffy thing out of there [referring to the microphone at the end of the long boom pole] we don't want anything scaring off this bird. Harry, you walk with the kid, keep a sharp look out, and protect the youngster if it attacks.' Appropriately he assumed a position at the rear as far away from the ensuing battle as possible. Almost in formation, the entourage strode to the park.

I'm looking dead ahead. Without warning this black and white missile is suddenly hurtling towards us; like that damn rocket at the start of the last Bond movie, it's coming straight for the little guy at my side. 'Look out!' and I pull the young lad against my thigh for protection. The bird flashes past. The tips of one wing brush the hand that buries the boy's head in my moleskins. Our magpie pulls out of the low-level strafing run, banks hard over to port and launches itself for a second onslaught. Wings folded back like a miniature F-111 in attack mode, the bird swoops down yet again. This time it is the beak that almost grabs a tuft of the child's hair, and he's gone. Back to a tall eucalypt at the far end of the park. He warbles a defiant call and turns his back on us lesser humans.

I'm shaking, the kid's shaking and his dad is patently worried. 'He's OK,' I announce with relief. We retreat to some cover of low-growing shrubs to consider the next move.

'Did you get that? Did you get it?' screams a totally ecstatic CB, because let's be honest, it was really real!

'No, mate, sorry we missed the lot, didn't get the camera rolling in time.'

'You didn't get it rolling!!!' The Dr Evil persona replaced the placid CB and he choked on the last few words of frustration. 'I told you twenty metres back to be ready.'

'Yeah, sorry, mate,' droned the camo, 'could we try it again?'

The look on Dr Evil's face should have been enough. No, we were definitely not going to try that stunt again. Got to give it to the doctor, though, nothing had been forgotten on this trip.

'Harry? Could we try out the props we brought?'

In a planning session some time prior to our departure we'd concluded that subjecting the young fella to more than one experience with this rotten bird could be too traumatic and downright irresponsible. 'So why not use a dummy,' had been an almost instant suggestion from us both. At great expense we had borrowed a child store dummy from the costume department of Channel Seven, and had the props carpentry team make us up a crude sort of billycart device. By simply attaching some 100 metres of rope we could tow the contraption across the park. Only one problem remained: the dummy was twice the size of our young martyr.

'There's no way the bird will go for that, it's too darn big,' I explained to the still frustrated producer.

'Can we chop it in half?'

I thought it was worth a try so we disassembled the whole shebang, removing the legs and all else below waist level. The hair and eye colour matched those of our subject and we had borrowed a shirt too. So the upper torso of this rather scantily clad dummy soon sat screwed and bolted to the centre of our four-wheeled contraption. The rope was laid out in a straight line. It was just a matter of reeling it in, and the vehicle and its ridiculous passenger made their way slowly and somewhat shakily over the uneven terrain of the park towards the bushes behind which we were hiding.

Sometimes lady luck is on your side. It was the very jerkiness of the whole procession that attracted the bird's attention and once again he swooped in to attack. This time the camo did have things right. We watched from our cover as the cranky black and white scoundrel darted in and out, pecking at the glass eyes and pulling at the hair. This was one mean maggie. Take after take rolled onto the camera's tape. The maggie came back for more and eventually we had enough footage 'in the can' to make it a good day.

Magpies like this can be very dangerous and the really aggressive ones, intent on protecting their territory, have to be relocated to areas far away. And that would be the fate of this guy.

Somehow trips to Queensland have always been a trifle hazardous. Very often it's the weather. It can be stinking hot (particularly to a Tasmanian). Like the day I foolishly suggested that perhaps a house call to the hills outside the city might provide a slightly cooler atmosphere. Hell's bells, the temperature on the back verandah when the crew arrived was 46 degrees Celsius. It was to be a surprise and there's no doubt the lady of the house got quite a shock when yours truly appeared around the corner. This poor dog of theirs was terrified of the ride-on lawn mower. We filmed at dusk, and by then the temperature was still in the high thirties. My guess is the dog had been hit by a flying stone from the mower at some stage, because it certainly wasn't the noise. Not an easy one to fix. It's hard for dogs to conquer genuine fear.

Then there was the guinea fowl that thought it was a dog. What a hell of a trip that was. All the way to Gympie in the middle of the worst floods for a decade. Roads closing all around us, still we ploughed on. We'll get there, I thought, but will we ever get back? We managed both. This poor bird had been brought up from a chick with only an old blue cattle dog for company. At the best of times guinea fowl are a somewhat flighty bird, being a native of the African plain, they live on the ground and wander about in large noisy groups, only to fly up in the air whilst emitting the most atrocious din at any sign of danger. Birds are simple creatures. Much less complex than dogs and cats. Their main claim to fame is 'imprinting' on the first thing they see after hatching from the egg. This bird thought it was a dog, and the poor old dog was to this bird what it thought all guinea fowls looked like. Talk about mixed up!

If the poor hound ever disappeared for more than a few seconds the distraught bird would start flapping about all over the place, calling and screeching for all its worth.

So how do you fix this one? Thank heavens in town we found a furniture store and purchased two long mirrors. These were set up opposite one another with about a metre in between. It was then just a matter of coaxing the poor old heeler to walk between the mirrors. Once the bird followed the dog through this reflective maze, suddenly there were myriad uncles and cousins staring out from the surrounding glassware.

The startled bird flew in the air, turned a triple somersault, and landed upside down in the midst of a hundred or so of its relations, all of whom also seemed to be in some state of disarray. Finally after several displays of aggression, the dust settled and the bird became a bird, though I still think he carries a torch for that very patient old cattle dog.

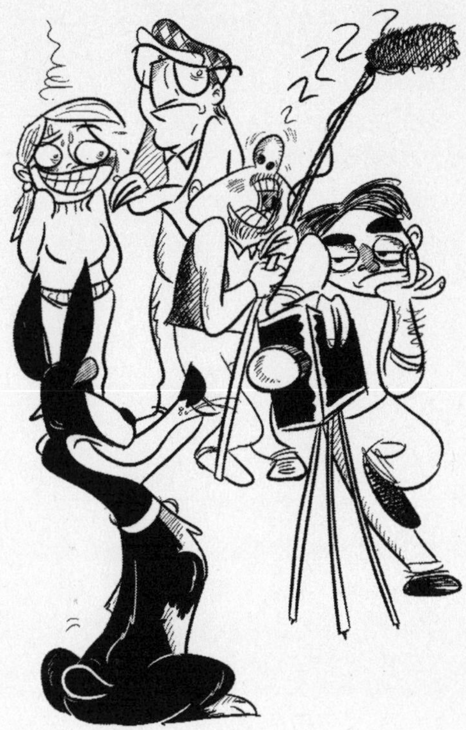

More TV House Calls

17

Top End Teasers

Over the last couple of years we at 'Harry's Practice' have literally spread our wings, just the turn of phrase you would expect from a vet who is crazy about birds anyhow. Darwin, Alice Springs, Adelaide, Perth, even Surfers Paradise have become part of our territory. Stories from the Top End always have a totally different flavour. It seems to someone who's spent nearly half his veterinary career only slightly north of the Antarctic that any temperature approaching 30 degrees must surely constitute life in a boiler room, not to mention the humidity. As soon as I step out of the confines of our air-conditioned Tarago, the spectacles instantly mist over and I find myself groping around in some sort of imagined fog for the gear buried in the back of the van. Still, you get used to it, I suppose.

The people are real characters, great, with a totally different attitude to life, to their animals and to us as a film crew. After all, not too many programs like ours really do take to the road, and I mean that in the true sense of the word. Darwin was quite an experience, I'd never seen the place before. Sure, you are aware of the myriad tropical diseases that your patients are likely to encounter in such a different environment, but strangely enough it's the same old situation that rears its head time and time again, regardless of where you are.

'My dog keeps chewing the tops off all me damned sprinklers. The bloody mangoes is all dyin'. A woman can't make a dollar.' She was an American ex-pat, came to visit the place some ten years ago, fell in love with it, bought a mango plantation and just never left. Home was a simple fibro and flyscreen netting enclosure, more like an upmarket carport than a house. Half the place had flooring, the other half had dirt. She lived with two dogs, one an old heeler cross and the other an impudent ten-month-old bull terrier cross God knows what. Half the dogs that seemed to inhabit the town were of similar breed, my guess is they're universally referred to as pig dogs. As ugly as the things they're meant to go out and hunt, scarred from left to right, most walk with some sort of a limp, many are missing an eye, a leg, or some other less functional part of their anatomy. They're a dog with character written all over their face and they're a dream to handle. To put it plainly their looks really belie their nature.

This perplexed lady with her southern American drawl was intent on explaining, in great detail, the growth cycle and water requirements of her mango trees. My training was more in veterinary science than horticulture, but suffice to say, in order to grow good mangoes it should rain when it doesn't, as well as rain when it does. 'You've got to water the bloody things in the winter, or they just don't set no bloody fruit.' (I wonder just how long it took her to acquire the great Australian adjective?) This young dog of hers was really out for a bit of a game.

'Get down here on the ground with me,' I said, lying flat on my belly to better survey the scene from the dog's point of view. That was a bit of an effort for her, she was quite a large lady and the upper part of her anatomy was supported almost entirely by a rapidly thinning masculine blue singlet, stuff was lollin' all over the place, I had to keep me eye on the dog, I can tell you.

'Look at all these things sticking up,' I said, pointing to the many little black stalks protruding some thirty to fifty centimetres above ground level. 'They look just like a lot of little flowers, don't they? When we were kids we'd walk home from school nipping the tops off all the seeding grasses and daisies along the way, wouldn't we? Anything within arm's reach we'd just grab it and for no other reason than it seemed the thing to do. A dog's no different to us. He'll grow out of it in time.'

'Yaarh,' she said, 'but all the bloody things will be dead by then.'

So it was solution time. To appreciate exactly why a dog is doing what you don't want it to do, put yourself in the place of the dog, both physically and mentally; it'll change your perception and make understanding canine behaviour all the more simple. You can't change a dog's normal behaviour – it's a matter of either removing the temptation altogether or putting a physical barrier between the dog and temptation. 'Two alternatives,' I said, 'either bury the sprinklers below ground level as soaker hoses or put a six-foot fence right around the place.' She opted for the latter.

Dogs really are very much like kids. Up to the age of ten months most are like children, beyond that they become young teenagers who go on to break windows, prang the family car and create all sorts of familial disruptions. Finally at the age of two and a half years, our canine friends have reached what we like to term social maturity – like our teenagers they've learnt to control their hormone surges, and have settled into a more normal and certainly more relaxed lifestyle. Regrettably, it takes most of our children another twenty years to accomplish the same ends, which is why Janine and I have got over twenty dogs and very few children.

Surprise house calls are something the whole crew enjoys. The thrill of the chase as it were, huddling behind the van getting all our gear together, testing the mikes, balancing the camera and we're off, creeping along one side of the building, turning the corner. 'There she is,' whispers the producer. 'Middle table in that archway, the brunette with her back to us, drinking coffee next to this bloke with the curly blond hair.' She didn't see us coming, he did, but kept his trap shut. A gentle tap on the shoulder. 'G'day, I'm Dr Harry, I'm here to have a look at this dog of yours that swims to Indonesia.' Well, she just about spilt the coffee all over him, me and herself. It always feels good when you pull off such an unexpected encounter.

This one was a bit of a setup, we knew she was out with her boss and not in the office, he was in on the setup and sure she could have the rest of the morning off to try to sort out this wretched dog. I love Staffies (Staffordshire bull terriers) and this was a rich red/fawn staffie bitch. 'We need to go down to the beach so you can see just exactly what she gets up to.'

'OK,' I said, 'how far is that?'

'Oh, about ten minutes' drive out of town.'

Have you ever seen a Darwin beach? At low tide it would take twenty minutes just to walk to the water's edge. Talk about sand – there are acres and acres of it and the water is very shallow for hundreds of metres out to sea. To put it simply, when the dog got to the beach and her owner removed the lead, the rotten little sod just set course due north and literally swam right out of sight.

'How'd you get her back?' I enquired.

'Most of the time she just won't come when I call. Sometimes she'll stay out for one or two hours, once she went missing for three days, but usually I have to wade out, grab her and haul her back in.'

'Isn't that a bit dangerous?'

''Tis, I suppose, there are stingers, sharks and probably the odd croc as well.'

'You didn't grow up around here did you?'

'No,' she said, 'I'm a bit of a Pom, can't you tell?'

And I thought the Poms were allergic to water. Not this girl, she loved this damned dog so much she'd have gone anywhere to retrieve it.

It's hard to be prepared for every eventuality but this time we were organised well in advance. Craig (a.k.a. CB), my intrepid producer, and I had discussed this problem at length before the trip.

'Get down to the fish market, son, buy me a big casting spool (you know, the plastic things) and about a hundred metres of good thick nylon line, about thirty kilograms breaking strain – that'll do the trick.' Being the good lad that he is, that's exactly what I was now unpacking from my bag of tricks.

'OK,' I advised, 'it's demonstration time. Take her down to the water's edge and show me what happens.' The dog took one look at the water and everything else became of no interest whatsoever; with a 'let me at it' expression on her face, the lead was off and the dog was gone, Indonesia, here I come!

'Try to call her back,' what a waste of time that was. 'Can you go and grab her before she's gone too far?' Wading out, my desperate owner collared the dog and dragged it, much to the dog's annoyance, out of the water and back up the beach.

'I'm gonna attach this thick fishing line to the dog's collar, I'll want you to let her go again and before she gets out too far we're going to yell "come". The biggest mistake most owners make is to use the dog's name while it's doing a runner. The dog thinks, "Last time I was doing a bolt they kept calling my name so it must be OK to keep running if they're calling my name this time." We've gotta change that by using a different command. "Come!" '

'Let 'er go.' The dog didn't need any translation – whoosh! And the canine Susie O'Neill was on her way north again. Some fifty metres had spooled from the caster in my left hand, it was time for action. 'Come!' I yelled, 'Come!' a second time and with my right index finger tensioned the rapidly unfurling line. 'Hell's bloody bells!' (that isn't exactly the turn of phrase I used at the time, it was slightly more expletive) as the nylon almost totally amputated the top of my right index finger. A twenty-kilo Staffie on the end of a simple nylon line without any gloves to help reel in the catch was a little stupid now I come to think about it. My finger was smoking, not a drop of blood, the burn of the line had been enough to cauterise every blood vessel within an inch or more of the wound. The dog stopped all right, it was then a matter of hauling in this canine catastrophe, by now my whole hand was aching, but the show must go on (my mother's words, not mine). So yours truly was charging up the beach, plastic caster under left armpit, right index finger in mouth, removing it only momentarily to issue another 'come' command to the dog, who was by now on the water's edge.

'Give her a treat . . . one of those things I gave you . . . just a bit, tell her she's a good girl.' By now, I'm eighty metres up the beach.

You learn by your mistakes. Naturally enough we had to repeat the whole procedure on at least another three occasions, so my dauntless camera crew could get enough shots to put the whole thing together into a story. It's a good technique for training dogs to come when they're called and very similar to that used by some of the better working-dog trainers down here in Tassie to school their young pups. But just be careful, folks, if you try this technique on your dog, make sure you've got a glove on at least one hand.

Alice Springs has, of course, sad memories for me, for that was the time when Rosie, our beloved Border Collie and working dog for so many years, left us forever. But there were other things so definitely Territorian that made for some happy memories mixed in with the sad.

For one the landscape is just totally different. The city is almost an oasis set in the middle of a countryside punctuated by dry creek beds, red and orange sands and jagged rocky outcrops. Their colour changes from purple to pink and ochre to grey depending on the angle of the sun, and from every and any direction the same formation takes on a completely different perspective. It's a wild land, almost an abandoned land – forgotten perhaps, sleeping maybe, but certainly so totally captivating that it beckons you back like some hypnotic drug. Set against this incredible background was a dog who simply liked collecting bottles and there were plenty of those around the Alice. But, folks, don't get the wrong idea, I'm not talking about the brown ones with long necks, I'm talking soft drink bottles, milk bottles, you name it. If it's plastic, the dog had to have it.

This dog resembled most of the other dogs about the place, cattle dog crossed with – well, your guess is as good as mine. Red in colour, spotted all over and covered with dust that disguised what little white may have been present. His home was a date farm. His owners grew date palms and harvested the dates to be sold both fresh and preserved in one form or another. The place was open to visitors day in and day out, but the dog was proving to be a real hazard for the owners. Things are pretty hot in the Alice and everyone knows that dehydration can kill, hence the need to drink plenty.

The picture is something like this. In walks a busload of tourists, some half a dozen or more carry water or soft drink in a plastic bottle dangling from one hand or the other, the dog lies in wait, springing his ambush when the unwary group is some ten or fifteen metres beyond his lair. Rushing in from behind like a canine purse-snatcher, he grabs the most grabbable bottle and is gone into the distance, his dusty hide providing genuine camouflage in this familiar terrain. When well out of sight he chews and gnaws at the bottle until it's broken, drinks the contents as they spill and then carts the empty off to his nest.

'You've got to be kidding, a nest, he's got a nest, this I've gotta see.' Sure enough that's what the dog had, just like a hairy four-legged bowerbird, this dog had amassed some thirty or forty mangled and flattened bottles in a large shallow depression under a tree behind the family home. This was his home, he slept on them, played on them, rearranged them, collected more, dispensed with some and generally found the whole episode not only amusing, but completely fulfilling. How do you explain something like this?

First of all, you try a few experiments. Different shaped bottles, with different contents, water, milk, soft drink, you name it. Cardboard containers, even the odd glass one just to judge the reaction, but it was plastic, folks, just plastic that this dog loved. The whole thing had become a game, possibly encouraged initially by the owners' amusement at the dog's behaviour, but it was now a very normal part of the daily routine. When dogs, particularly working dogs, are bored, they invent their own games.

To solve a problem like this it's a matter of diverting the dog's attention to something else other than the tourists' thirst quenchers. We used frisbees and the dog took to them almost instantly. With patience I'm sure we can convert this character into a frisbee collector and not a bottle pincher. But why the nest? Quite honestly, I dunno, perhaps he'd heard somewhere about a waterbed, but then being a conservation-conscious canine he opted to have the bed without the water. Well, that's my theory, you come up with a better one.

No story about the Territory would be complete without camels. So there we were, crack of dawn at the local Alice camel farm. They ran safaris outta town to all places of interest. I've ridden them once or twice. The motion is certainly much like riding in a dinghy, probably hence the name 'ships of the desert', but the seat I find is so terribly broad, it's like doing a half-splits all day. From an environmental point of view, they're a great animal, big, broad feet to cover the ground with minimal impact, thick eyelids and eyelashes to keep out the dust and a ready-made supply of both water and energy stored in their hump as fat!

There were two patients, one with a large growth on its nictitating membrane (third eyelid). Yep, we've only got two, but most of the animal kingdom has got an extra one. Sun and sun alone is usually responsible for the development of these tumours, which can usually be removed under general anaesthesia. The difficulty is getting the camel to hold still long enough to get a good look at the damned thing. A few appropriately chosen words of Arabic will usually get them to lie down, but holding that big head in the one place for any more than a few seconds takes a superhuman effort. They are the world's greatest sooks, hate pain and hate any sort of physical intrusion.

His mate had an equally minor problem, a lump about half the size of a tennis ball attached to the skin between both front legs. It was a pretty fair bet that this was simply caused by a foreign body like a grass seed or a thorn. Removal would have been easy, but the moment the camel even caught sight of a needle he was up and outta there before one drop of local anaesthetic even entered the tissues around the lump. Legs, feet, head, handler and Dr Harry seemed to be flying in all directions. The noise was deafening; it's a sort of eerie mournful wail that would seem to suggest medieval torture was about to be inflicted instead of twenty-first century surgery. Who would have thought an animal that'd put up with so much in its natural environment would turn to jelly at even the thought of pain. We ran out of time, planes wait for no man, so I referred the problems to one of my colleagues in town.

The landscape, the people, the very different animals will one day bring Dr Harry and his film crew back to the Top End.

18

It's Got Me Licked

I love the city of Adelaide, Colonel Light certainly got things right when he designed the layout. The whole thing being in a grid pattern is easy to navigate. The streets are wide and majestic, the older parts have been preserved and the new parts buzz with life and alfresco eating and drinking. On a trip away you only get to enjoy this side of life after the day's work is done. Most of our visits take us to the country or at least the suburbs, and you'd be surprised how many people still think that our surprise house calls are setups.

To prove the point we were joined by the local newspaper. 'Seven o'clock in the morning!' exclaimed the not-too-enamoured young journalist who was to accompany us the next morning.

'Yep, seven o'clock in the morning, meet us at the hotel, and don't be late, we need to be knocking on doors at 7.30 before people go to work.'

There is always a shortlist of possible visits and the idea is to have one main one and a couple of backups if the first one falls over. A chook that thinks it's a dog sounds like a good story. The chook sleeps with the dog, it grew up with the dog, we know that much. Seven-thirty, right on cue. Knock on the door, no answer, not even a barking dog, I could see the chooks over the side gate. Seven-thirty in the morning and no one's home, you'd better believe it, get out of there in a hurry before the neighbours wake up to what's going on. We'll try it again tomorrow.

It wasn't to be our day, the next two were not home either, that's the worst strike-out we'd experienced – number four coming up and we're scraping the bottom of the barrel. By this time I'm sure our young scribe believed things were genuine, but so far there was nothing to write about. Time is now about 9.30 – fingers crossed, here we go.

'G'day, I'm Dr Harry and I'm here to look at your licking dog.'

She was pretty surprised, not too much of the ooh or ah, but genuinely shocked that I'd come. To catch a lady in her dressing gown at 9.30 in the morning is probably more embarrassing than shocking.

'So what's the problem with this dog of yours?'

'Well, Dr Harry, he licks everything.'

'What do you mean he licks everything?'

'Well, he licks the furniture, all around the doors, the carpet, the lino and people as well.'

'OK, why don't you go and get dressed, we'll set up a few lights and try to catch the dog doing a bit of his old tongue trick.'

Ten minutes later she was back, the patient was a cocker spaniel about eight years old and blue roan in colour. He had a mate, also a cocker, this one a black, and a lot younger. The good lady made us all a cup of tea and we sat around the dining table waiting for the dog to do his thing. Twenty minutes passed, the dog sat there, looking at us. 'Ignore the dog, don't look at the dog.' It didn't matter what we did or said. The dog just sat there, looking at us.

'Does he lick all the time?'

'Oh yes, he never stops licking.'

'But he hasn't done anything, he's just sitting there.'

'Yes.'

'I know this can happen sometimes, when a whole group of strangers comes into your home it tends to upset things a bit, perhaps we should just go out and leave the cameraman here to get the pictures.' We did. Strolling around the garden, my client explained that Simon, being the dog's name, of course, had been doing this licking with increasing frequency over the last two years and she'd tried all sorts of horrible goo painted on the furniture and the doors. But after all, 'You can't paint it on the visitors,' and it didn't seem to work anyhow.

Fifty minutes had passed when we walked back into the room, there was good old Simon, totally unmoved by the whole situation, simply staring up at my cameraman with a look of complete bliss or perhaps total lack of interest, I don't know which.

'Has he done anything, mate?'

'Harry, apart from breathing, nothing at all.'

We sat again. The producer was getting anxious.

'How much longer, Harry, before this dog licks?'

'Let's give it another ten minutes,' I suggested.

'He must start licking soon,' my now somewhat anxious client blurted.

Silence reigned!

It was now well over the hour.

'That's it,' I said, 'we're out of here.' The producer breathed a sigh of relief, the journalist wondered what the heck she was going to write about and all the soundo could talk about was what he was going to have for lunch.

'He must lick soon, he will lick, I tell you he licks, you don't believe me, do you?'

'Look,' I tried to explain, 'this is television, I believe you, I believe the dog does lick, but we have to see the dog lick or we don't have a story.'

'He will lick, if you just give him another minute.'

'Sorry, it's been an hour and a quarter and I haven't even seen him lick his lips, let alone anything else.'

She wasn't happy, I was disappointed, but that's the way it goes. The next one was down at McLaren Vale and if that one fell over too then we could always drown our sorrows at one of the local vineyards.

The lady we were calling on at McLaren Vale was surprised, in fact, so surprised she'd forgotten she'd even written to me. 'Who are you?'

'I'm Dr Harry.'

'What are you doing here?'

'I'm here because you wrote to me.'

'I did? . . . Oh yes, you're the vet man on TV.'

After an intro like that, things just had to get better. Her dog was frightened of the bird-scaring devices that were used at harvest time around the many vineyards of the area. They were gas operated 'guns' that fired off loud noises on an irregular basis to keep the birds away from the grapes. Quite a lot of dogs have genuine noise phobias and these are made so much worse because of the volume and sheer mechanical impact that the force of the explosion produces. We had to hire one for the afternoon to demonstrate the problem, as they were not in use at that time of year.

One was set up in my client's front garden and the dog showed all the predictable fear responses associated with the weaponry. We came equipped with all the right desensitising machinery. A CD with every bang and boom invented by mankind, which we played back to the dog in ever-increasing volume, and then reinforced our total disregard for the event by throwing a party – fancy hats and all. This tends to send a message to the dog that there is really nothing to worry about because we're not worried, so why should it be. Dogs look to us for some sort of message about how to behave and if we as owners are sympathetic to dogs that exhibit these kinds of phobias, they become intensified and ingrained as part of the dog's behaviour. This dog needed medication as well, and hopefully she's feeling a lot better come the next grape harvest.

I'm constantly asked if these surprise calls are really genuine. The answer, as you've seen, is yes. If they are not, then they do not go to air. There was a lady in Melbourne who, in spite of several early morning calls, we were unable to catch at home. The problem was she had a little silkie cross that every time she drove off to work, would go ballistic and start shredding the curtains in the lounge room window. This sounded like a case of separation anxiety, and would be worth filming. After a bit of investigation, our trusty producer was able to discover that she didn't work Fridays.

We are at the ready. It's 7.30 a.m. and I'm knocking on the door. The lady who answers my knock is anything but surprised. She looks like she's just stepped off the cover of a fashion magazine. Not a hair out of place, glossy red lipstick and matching nail varnish. That dress must've set her back a pretty penny. She feigned surprise. I glanced at the producer. We were more stunned than she was. Who looks like this at 7.30 in the morning, unless, of course, you're expecting visitors!

After a quick conference we decided to go ahead anyhow,

and use the story not as a surprise, but as a normal house call.

'Tell me exactly what the dog does,' I asked.

'Well, when I leave to go to work in the car, little Timmy starts jumping up and down at the window. He's scratched all the paint and torn some of the curtains.' I could see the evidence right enough.

'We need to see little Timmy do his stuff,' I advised, 'could you go through your normal leaving-for-work routine and we'll film what happens?'

She obliged, and backed the car out and drove away.

'The dog did nothing,' I informed the good lady on her return.

'That's because you're all here,' she retorted. That may very well be true. Often animals don't perform when we're around. So we all went with her except the cameraman. Once again same result!

'It's the camera fella!' she exclaimed. 'He'll have to go as well.'

Rod set up the camera on a low tripod and we all left.

What did we see on our return? A few shots of the dog wandering around, quietly sniffing the camera, and at the very end, a shot of the dog's underside as he emptied his bladder with some disdain all over the lens!

'I'm sorry, we just can't do the story. The dog did none of the things you said he would.'

'What! You're not going to put little Timmy and me on television after I've spent all this money on my hair and nails!' Gotcha! Some surprise, eh! No, we didn't. Sure I sat with her for twenty minutes and explained what she could do to solve the problem. A man wasted his breath!

What amazed me for a long time is that children are never really surprised to see me.

It's a Sydney suburb, and I'm calling to surprise a family with budgie troubles. There in the street, right in front of the house are a couple of kids playing.

'Are you Tony Watson?' I whispered to the elder of the two.

'Yes, hello, Dr Harry,' he whispered back totally unfazed, 'and this is my sister Rebecca.'

'Where is your mum?'

'She's up in the kitchen doing some cooking.'

'OK. Don't tell her I'm here, and we'll sneak up and surprise her.'

Halfway up the front steps it all goes wrong.

'Mum – Dr Harry is here!' screams young Rebecca. There's an answering scream from the kitchen where Mum stands, aghast, her hands covered in flour.

We do the story, and at the end I ask something that for all the time I've been knocking on doors has puzzled me.

'Why weren't your children surprised to see me?'

'It's simple,' she replied, 'you're a bit like Father Christmas. They write to him every year and he comes. They write to you. Of course you'll come.'

Father Christmas, eh. Never thought of that.

19

Queensland Originals

One thing about getting out of the city is that we meet some real characters. Travelling round the back blocks of North Queensland was no exception. Surprising people at home or in their workplace is great, but often just finding the place is the hardest part of the job. The directions on this occasion were vague, to say the least. Our researcher had done her best but couldn't get exact details, as we wanted to catch this lot out.

What we did know was they owned a fish and yabby farm and that it was a good forty minutes' drive out of town. The local garage is always good for directions.

'Yeah. Well, you gotta get over the other side of the river, but the bridge is out [we knew that much], so youse'll 'ave to go right at the big depot down in the town, look out for all the cane trucks and trains 'cos it's right in the middle of harvest. Go over that low culvert, keep on for about . . . Hang on, is that Dr Harry in there? G'day, Dr Harry!'

'And from there . . .' went on Steve.

'Oh yeah, sorry, yeah, take the left fork and as you climb the hill you'll see the nets and everything over the big ponds.' Steve swallowed hard and prayed he'd remember. Petrina, the producer, had made a few notes; between us we'd get there.

Just as she said, as we crested the hill there were the nets, but no house. That figures: if you take the right fork you get to the house. Andre is a whiz kid at U-turns. Up the right fork and a slow drive past the place. Problems right from the start. There are two houses. Which one? The dirt road is wide, complete with massive table drains on each side to deal with the tropical downpours. There's red dust all over everything. Petrina hops into the driver's seat. I'm in the front, alongside her, black bag ready to go. Steve on sound and Andre with camera are hooked up and 'standing rigidly by'. Slowly the Tarago creeps up over the hill.

'Pull up on the wrong side of the road,' whispers Andre, 'Steve and I'll hop out and Harry, you just go for it, we'll be right behind.'

It is 7.45 Sunday morning. Petrina applies the brakes and I'm out and heading straight for the big house, oblivious to the melee behind me. Steve and Andre, in their hurry to get out, both go for opposite sides of the car. An impossible manoeuvre as they are connected by a three-metre black audio cable. Petrina spins round to help untangle the situation and places her left elbow squarely on the horn, which shatters the early morning calm for miles around. Andre is yelling to me, 'Wrong house . . . wrong house!', but I'm striding towards the more lived-in of the two dwellings anyhow. Then from out of nowhere comes this three-year-old child.

'Hello, Dr Harry . . . the sick lamb is over here in the paddock.' I'm dumbfounded.

'Where is your mum?' I asked, seeking to delay things a little so the rest of my lot can catch up.

'She's up inside.'

'Can you call her?'

'Mummy, can you come out here for a minute?' commands this unbelievably articulate youngster in bare feet and a simple cotton dress. Mum appears on the verandah, sees the camera, the sound boom and me. She instantly screams. Now the whole valley is awake. Talk about a surprise! Finally calm is restored, but only temporarily. Andre's got about half of what happened and poor old Steve, he's trying to retrieve his audio lead from the dog! A bull terrier who happens to be part of the family as well. Finally everybody gets the shots and the sounds they want, Petrina's happy and we go looking for the lamb.

According to my information this lamb is supposed to be lame. Well, that it may be, but a lamb with three legs is a better bet than an ageing vet with two. After three failed attempts we finally gather the mob of sheep and assorted lambs in one corner of the paddock. There are around a dozen of each. My patient is easy to spot, he's a part-bred Suffolk with brownish feet and face, a couple of months old. But the way he moves, you'd never pick him as lame. Mum's yelling, the kids are yelling (yes, we've been joined by another three-year-old, who's on a sleepover) and no one is taking any notice of me! They make a dash to the right.

'Block them!' I yell . . . they do. Then they break left, and it's all or nothing. With a dive that George Greegan would be proud of, the lamb comes to ground wrapped safely in the arms of myself. Vets in the country need to be fairly athletic; sad to relate my best days are behind me.

Everyone's excited. We carry the lamb back to some shelter near the house. The sun is already doing its very best to cook us all. A quick examination reveals that the poor little fella has broken his elbow. According to 'Mum' he got himself caught up in a roll of fencing wire and that's how the damage occurred. The elbow is a complicated joint and without the benefit of X-ray I can only feel that it's broken in about three places and already starting to heal. The outlook is good, but the joint will be permanently stiff once healing is complete. On top of that there is an open wound with all the worry of fly strike and infection. This we can treat. Sounds quick and easy, eh? It is, but add a three-year-old and a producer, and what should have been a three-minute examination and two-minute treatment turns into an hour and a half. For ninety minutes I restrain this lamb so all the right shots are taken and the story can be told by my young superstar. When it's all over, the lamb can go back to its mum, who's been bleating constantly the whole time. It won't get up. It cannot stand. It just lies there, and it looks like lying there for keeps!

In animal behaviour we talk about a situation called learned helplessness. Simply explained, it means when an animal tries to resist something and finds it impossible to overcome the problem, it finally just gives up and its body collapses. This was what we had here! This lamb is going to croak. Yep, it's headed for the big muster in the sky. All except the poor vet on duty (me) are up on the verandah, eating cream sponge and drinking tea. I'm trying to reverse the situation with glucose drenches and cortisone injections. Stalling for time to give my drugs a chance to work, we all tour the yabby ponds and the fish farm. (Fish farming is a worry. You go to bed at night and they all look fine; get up the next morning and half are dead. That's the way it goes.) Finally, after some vain attempts at standing and almost an hour's encouragement the little bugger gets to his feet and wanders off to find Mum. Whew! Later that day I get a message, 'Mum and son both doing well.' Thanks. I really appreciated that!

Surprising people is still the best buzz on television, especially when you've trekked through North Queensland rainforest to find them. The letter was signed by 'Winka'. She had a problem with this new draught horse filly she'd bought and her mule. The mule couldn't stand the sight of the horse! After driving through acres of cane the road finally turns up the mountain, and into a dirt track! Even in good conditions it would be difficult to pass and impossible to overtake. At its end are three properties. None have numbers. We only have a name. None have signs either. 'Eenie, meenie' springs to mind, but hang on, this one looks likely – besides, the mob next door have just driven off to church. There's an electric fence around the whole joint. These must be ten-acre blocks. The gate is also blocked by electric tape.

'Relax, guys, it's off.' The wet strand of grass in my hand fails to conduct any current. The drive is steep, very, very steep, and it's hard work for Andre and Steve with all their gear, when from out of nowhere this dune buggy appears over the top of a hill, headed straight for us. The thing is a converted 'Vee Dub' with a bearded gent at the controls and a youngster of about ten in the rear.

'No brakes,' he yells as the thing slides past in a beautiful four-wheel drift and comes to rest against a large eucalypt.

'We're looking for Winka,' spouts Petrina.

'She's up there. You'll find her at the house.'

'Don't tell her we're coming.'

'Don't worry about that, lady, this old girl probably won't make it up the hill before you do. Bloody thing's stuck in second gear, and we can't turn her around. Can we, boy?'

At the top of the hill we see the house. Washing's on the line, there are animals everywhere, but no Winka. A full-frontal approach seems the go.

'Just go for the front door,' says Andre as we cross the front yard.

'Where is the damn thing? I can't see any door,' I whisper. But I can see a window that's covered in flyscreen and the back of a woman just inside it. She's on the phone. We creep up. I open the screen quietly, tap her on the shoulder, she turns around and . . .

'G'day. Are you Winka?' She screams, and then screams into the phone as well. I even get to talk to her friend to assure her that it really is Doctor Harry!

The house is set atop a hill in the middle of a rainforest. They built the lot themselves from scratch, using only local timber. I've never seen flame cedar before. Tongues of fire seem to leap out from the newly cut surface of the logs. It makes beautiful furniture, but the sawdust is extremely toxic. Talk about tranquillity. This is it. The farm is something else, there are all sorts of animals here: chickens, turkeys, ducks, guinea fowl, kangaroos, and goats all scrabble round for a bit of tucker. Then, of course, there's the troublesome mule. We meet every one of them, sort out the equine situation, and eat marvellous homemade biscuits, with real tea, only just before the kangaroo scoffs the lot. As a final gesture a bald cocky makes an appearance, gently touching my skin with his poor deformed beak. He has only three feathers. Like so many of his fellow sufferers, his life will be short, as he has an untreatable viral disease. Sure, he looks like a blue Woolworths chicken, but that's the bird's natural skin colour, it's not that he's feeling the cold.

Winka writes every now and then, sends a little gift and keeps us up to date on how things are going with her new baby (the horse, of course) and the mule. It is people like this that make the whole job just so worthwhile.

20

Porcine Paradise

House calls of course take us all over Australia, and my native Tasmania is no exception. Once again it was Craig at the helm. There were, it seems, these two pigs that had suddenly developed terrible problems with their skin. We wouldn't have to go too far out of Hobart and this one sounded like a challenge. Stories like this have definite appeal, it's a chance to look at a very different animal and it isn't every day you get called out to a couple of pigs. What a pretty spot the farm was set on, as so many on the island are. The house was built quite high up on some very hilly ground and the verandah had a fabulous view of the D'Entrecasteaux channel and beyond.

'The pigs are over here,' explained the lady of the house, 'we've had them penned up for the last ten days.'

'Where did you get them?' I enquired as we walked towards the rather primitive pigpen.

'Oh, we bought them only recently from an indoor piggery.'

You didn't have to be a genius to work this one out. They were white pigs, suddenly exposed to the savage Tassie summer sun, made worse yearly by the yawning hole in the ozone layer. The poor devils were sunburnt.

'Good, Harry,' says Craig in his usual manner, 'we can all see that. What do you propose doing about it?'

It's never any good simply rushing into things. By now it was getting on a bit in the afternoon, even allowing for the twilight that would follow. Things were not quite as easy as they looked, so the owner and I planned just how we could catch one or both pigs inside their flimsy run. The enclosure was about forty metres long and four or five wide. The fences were constructed from very poorly anchored sheep and lamb fencing wire, supported with a series of somewhat teetering metal star pickets. It all looked a bit on the temporary side to me. Very temporary! This won't hold much, I thought, better to look for something more solid.

'We can catch them in the shed if I put some feed in there,' suggested the ever-helpful owner. Ah yes, folks, sounds easy, but the pigs had other ideas. The very thought that now there were an extra group of four humans clustered around their home aroused in their porcine brains some sense of foreboding. The same sense was developing in mine too!

One of the two finally ventured into the shed. The owner blocked off one exit and I blocked the other. Funny how none of the film crew ever wants to get involved! It was up to her young son and us. Like a champagne cork from a bottle, the rapidly reddening porker dashed for the door, straight between the owner's legs, completely bowling her over. It took one look at me, decided freedom was the only alternative, and with a squeal of delight promptly nosed its way under the fence and shot through into the distance! I was dead right about the fences. The second pig, having been a passive observer of the whole episode, also decided that capture was the last thing on its mind and in less than a second joined her mate. What a great start to the story! Now instead of having two patients neatly cooped up in a run, we had two feral baconers galloping for all their worth around five acres, and two pigs on the go can really move!

For nearly two hours the owner, her children and I exhausted ourselves physically and mentally in an effort to catch these rogue animals. Would anyone help? Not likely, they were all too busy laughing as the lot of us clutched vainly for a grasp of the escapees.

'Better give it away, Harry,' advised our illustrious producer. The cameraman was looking rather anxiously towards the setting sun.

'We're going to run out of light, mate,' they advised in unison.

'I'm not finished yet . . . Give me another half an hour,' I pleaded in between breaths. This was hard work.

Suddenly the tide turned our way. Right down the end of the long flimsy pig run and just outside it lay the absorption pit for the septic tank. The ground was soggy, black and stinking with the smell of effluent. A perfect pig wallow. Just the ideal spot for them to want to lie in. Let's face it, by now they were as hot as all of us. Slowly but surely we guided the pair of them over to the area. Ah! Heaven! Well, that is, if you're a pig. They soon started nosing about, as pigs do, turning over the slimy inky mess with their muscular noses. It was easy digging and the feel and smell of the mud was obviously to their liking. This was the opportunity to strike. Closer and closer we crept in a crude attempt to hold them in place.

'See if you can hold them in there and I'll grab one,' I advised with a confident tone. Slowly I advanced, but once I got within a metre of my quarry they were up and gone. So near yet so far. Perhaps we should have whispered our plans, or maybe pigs can lip-read.

It was worth another try, at least. Everyone was tired, particularly me. This would be the last throw of the dice. Time was running out. The two renegades finally returned to the wallow and commenced digging with a vengeance. Just wait, I thought, till one of them puts her whole head under the mud, she won't see me coming. The moment arrived, and so did I!

'Gotcha!!!' as my right hand locked around one very slimy hind foot. 'Gotcha,' and she was up in the air and into my arms.

World War Five exploded. You have never heard so much yelling and screaming in all your life. Once you get a pig's legs off the ground, the animal just about goes ballistic. Was the cameraman going to come to me? Was anyone going to help? No way. They're splitting their sides laughing. So on top of all the chasing I had to lug this twenty kilos of slippery, struggling bacon all the way back up to where the intrepid crew was waiting. Ever tried to talk over the top of a squealing pig? All you could do was to speak whenever the pig stopped to draw breath. It was the most disjointed sound session ever recorded. The noise of the pig's cries for help blew the limiter on the soundo's machine. He had to go into manual mode. By the end of my dissertation on sunburn and its prevention I think both his ears were internally haemorrhaging.

It all ended with the young son aiming to throw a bucket of medicated wash all over the pig, but in all the wrestling and screaming he got a trifle confused and emptied most of the contents over me! Ah well, all in a day's work, but I'm pleased to report that house calls to pigs have been placed very much on the back burner.

21

Duck Dilemmas

Somehow or other, ducks and I have some strange sort of affinity. Perhaps it goes back to my early childhood where the very first pet that I was permitted to keep was a duckling called 'Squeaker' about whom I have written elsewhere.

There is a wide assortment of duck breeds. The Muscovy, perhaps the most popular breed, is strangely enough not a duck at all. Sure it may look like a duck, but it has no 'quack', it lays only seasonally and the eggs take thirty-five days to hatch. Exactly one week longer than a true duck! The breed hisses like a goose and is probably far more like this larger cousin than its general demeanour would have us believe. When we talk ducks this fella is on the outer. Let's concentrate on the Khaki Campbells, the Pekins, the mallards, the Rouens, the Cayugas, the Aylesburys, and the Orpingtons, that'll do for starters.

The study of bird behaviour is certainly in its infancy. Much has been learnt about the way dogs, and to a lesser degree cats, interact with one another and with us human beings. As for birds, to which large family ducks belong, one could probably write our current state of knowledge on a bus ticket! Analysing bird behaviour is like untangling a spider's web without getting any of the sticky stuff on your fingers. A house call to a misbehaving duck is therefore something of a challenge, and that's putting it mildly!

Firstly there was the duck that the owner thought was

attacking the dog. Not too far out of Hobart in the south of Tasmania, a delightful family was the proud owner of a pair of Indian runners. This breed originated in the East Indies and is characterised by the way they look and move. Standing bolt upright like a penguin, having very little meat on their chests, and with long skinny necks, they run like the clappers when frightened, resembling an army of toy soldiers beating a hasty retreat.

As I've said before, the golden rule with any house call is if we don't get to actually see the behaviour then we simply do not have a story. After all, this is television. It is a visual medium and depends on pictures. We don't need to talk about it, we need to see it.

The family lived on a small farm that was dotted with fruit trees and clothed in a mantle of green from the recent rains. The man of the house was there to greet me on arrival.

'Morning, I'm Dr Harry, and I believe you have a duck problem of sorts,' that's the usual beginning to any story out on the road.

'Yes, we have. Our duck keeps attacking our English sheepdog.'

'Very interesting . . . could I see what happens?'

So out from under the house comes the poor long-suffering and by now somewhat perplexed-looking bearded Collie cross.

'I need to see exactly what happens, can you give me a demonstration?' I enquired. Yes, *he* could but the question always is: will the duck and the dog oblige? The owner walks down through the middle of his apricot orchard with the dog in close pursuit. From left of field this white projectile hurtles through the trees in pursuit of his hairy canine victim. The dog obviously knows from experience just what to expect and had long ago decided that surrender was the best course of action if ever confronted with a clone of Ferdinand from the film *Babe*. The dog drops to the ground. The duck, or more correctly the drake, whose sex I have been able to determine from its tail feathers, jumps on the dog.

'It's attacking Jessie,' the owner stammers with some feeling of guilt. By now the whole family is watching the proceedings from the sunroom window. The dog lay there on its belly seemingly unable to move. With one quick bite the whole contest would have been over, and with the amount of flesh on an Indian runner there would have been only two mouthfuls to swallow at the most.

'Let's leave them to it,' I suggested, as the drake ran from one end of the dog to the other, quacking and flapping his wings, 'and have a look around.' This we did, only to discover that over in one corner we had another duck, this one a female and sitting on a large clutch of eggs.

'Does he spend a lot of time over here with the female?' I enquired casting an inquisitive look toward the drake and the dog, still seemingly enjoying one another's company 100 metres away.

'Oh, yes, he stays fairly close to her all the time.' Further to that, the drake's seeming aggression to the dog had become far worse the moment the female started sitting, I was also informed. Was this then just a simple matter of the male of the species protecting his territory and primarily his mate? Well, sort of.

Ten minutes later and the damn duck, sorry, drake, is still at it. Running up and down the back of the dog, grabbing tufts of hair, jumping off and checking out the dog's ears. Climbing on again. More hair tugging interspersed with a copious amount of quacking and general nibbling of the skin. This is a bit more than the usual defence of territory routine! How do you explain in the nicest possible way to a young couple and their children that this drake of theirs is actually attempting to mate, yes, I said *mate*, with their dog. Are all drakes that blind? No, they are not. Are all drakes that randy? Yes, at the right time of year they most definitely are!

The Blue Mountains west of Sydney have always been a good hunting ground for 'Harry's Practice' stories, and they too have their fair share of duck problems. Enter a very large Pekin drake, named Henry. The only duck on the entire place, but causing more trouble than a whole flock of feathered females. This duck was owned by a couple who, deciding life in the city was not to their liking, moved to a small acreage in the rocky bushland that is so typical of the area. The house was a long bungalow style with a large glassed-in area to catch the best of the warm winter sun and the stunning views over the valley, which literally plunged from the back garden to a creek at its base. Sharing the household were a budgerigar and a cat, and this is precisely where the problem lay.

The budgerigar, being only a small bird and confined to what was a gargantuan cage considering the size of the occupant, posed no threat to either the cat or the duck. The bird was of quite stunning appearance being a Harlequin Pied, its body splashed with irregular patches of yellow and green, enhancing its ability to camouflage in the over-decorated cage. The cage and its occupant mainly spent daylight hours outside, on the barbecue table, the cage stuffed full of every wildflower and seeding grass his over-zealous owner could possibly ram inside. There was very little room left to fly. On top of this collection of feathers, flora and faeces sat Albert the cat. This was not just an accidental partnership between bird and its mortal enemy the cat, but rather something contrived and fostered by the lady of the house as a highly desirable relationship. The very presence of the cat deterred the advance and attack by any marauding scoundrels like currawongs and butcherbirds. The bird seemed totally undaunted by the presence of the cat and the cat seemed blissfully unaware of the mass that it sat above, principally because of the large carpet offcut that the owner had positioned atop the cage, separating the two.

The problem lay squarely with the duck. To get to his favourite spot in the sun Albert the cat had to negotiate a small area of paved courtyard between the back door and the barbecue setting. No more then ten metres at most, and this is where Henry would spring his trap, lying in wait just behind the twisted steel archway that supported an ancient climbing rose (this was the back door). There would be a rapid exchange of hisses and screams, most emanating from the now rapidly retreating Albert, who, being shown no mercy by Henry, was pursued inside the door and halfway down the hall of the house. Human intervention came to naught. The lady of the house stepping in to referee the stoush was summarily attacked from toe to ankle by the now seemingly rabid duck closing for the kill. Only recourse to the straw broom sent the protagonist into reverse. By now the cat was terrified and counted his days in the sun as being less and less likely as time went by. He had become so introverted as to require a human escort to cross what must have seemed like the battlefields of Flanders. In short, he had to be carried everywhere. The lady of the house had taken to wearing rubber boots as the ferocity of Henry's onslaught became directed at her since the feline adversary had seemingly joined the airborne group.

There's no doubt about it, this was the crankiest of all cranky drakes. He even went for me, taking a stranglehold on the trusty moleskins, till I retorted with a similar hold around Henry's neck! This is all about territory. Male ducks become very over the top when it comes to defending what they rightly or wrongly believe to be their territory. The only solution to a drake with these behaviour patterns is to lock him up. Henry now has his very own pen and Albert has found his place in the sun again.

Children are often the subject of attacks by wayward drakes and cockerels as well. It's all got to do with their size and the way they react to the onslaught. Filbert was some sort of a mallard cross. He lived with a veritable bevy of females. Four in all and was kept fairly busy making sure that the eggs they laid were fertile. The girls were all Pekins, or something vaguely like the breed, basically white in colour with flesh-coloured beak and feet. He, on the other hand, was resplendent in a suit of assorted shades of brown, a dash of white and that magnificent green that looks almost black and burnished when the sun hits it. They all happily shared an enclosure, surrounded by a low wire mesh fence, narrow gate and sporting their very own large converted fishpond in the centre.

Filbert was seemingly always on the warpath and the kids didn't make things any easier for themselves by always parading past the duck pen in bare feet! The sight of so many fat, wiggling worms presented five at a time was just too much for this rampant drake. He would fly at the wire in a desperate attempt to latch onto one or more. This, of course, as it often does with children, developed into a bit of a game. But as you often discover when working with animal problems, what starts out as a minor game ends up as a major problem. For all of his four or more kilos, Filbert was now a major problem.

When on the odd occasion he was let out of the pen for a spot of free grazing on the lawn, he reckoned anyone in sight was fair game, particularly if they were under the age of ten. This darn drake would line up his quarry like a sophisticated ground-to-air missile. First a step back, as if to measure his run, then commencing into aircraft taxi mode, as soon as the target appeared in view he would rattle down the make-believe runway, lift no more than a foot from the ground and rocket towards the target. In most instances he scored a direct hit. Accompanied by the soprano scream of yet another victim caught unprepared.

Desexing would be the only permanent answer to a problem like this but my clients opted for some further fencing modifications to give the drake a trifle more freedom and the children a darn sight more security when playing.

There is yet one more tale to tell about ducks, or rather drakes, and this one revolves round a surprise house call. It was in one of Melbourne's older suburbs, where the houses were built to last and the land on which they sit is just so much more substantial in size than the miserable building blocks of today. The house was two storeys, built from hefty sandstone blocks and the upper storey supported an ornate balcony. As with all surprises we cased the joint first, driving by slowly so the camera crew could suss out the lie of the land. I sat in the back seat with the morning paper held as close to my face as possible to prevent recognition. Satisfied that a straightforward walk up would be the go, the crew car was left around the corner and up we strode.

Pushing open the tall cast-iron front gate we literally fought our way through the piles of rubble and weeds that masqueraded as a front garden. Up just three wide sandstone steps stood the majestic front door. Hang on . . . it was one-third open!

'Do you think they've spotted us?' I queried Andre.

'No way, mate, just look at all that ornate stained glass . . . no one could see through that.'

The huge metal doorknocker landed on its contact plate with a clang that would surely wake everyone in the street. I swung it again. *Clang.g.g.g.*

'Yes, what do you want?' came a faint and timid voice from somewhere within the lower part of the house. I declined to reply.

'Listen, Andre, I'm going to shove this door right open and we're all going in . . . OK?' I whispered. He nodded and with that the huge door swung back on its hinges and we were in, striding down the entrance hall, past bedrooms spilling over with heaps of clothes, and other doors refusing to close from the cacophony of junk that lay behind them. All but tripping over the threadbare carpet as we turned the corner, there they were, mother and daughter, huddled together in their dressing gowns, shaking like leaves on an autumn poplar.

'Gee,' she stammered, 'we thought it was a home invasion!' Well, at 7.30 on a weekday morning I suppose one could. Time for my two ladies to get dressed and gather their senses before we tackle the problem.

'And what is the problem?' I asked.

'The drake keeps strangling the chook.' Yes, folks, that was it in a nutshell, and we couldn't wait to see a re-enactment.

On the whole, birds seldom let you down and this would be

no exception. Having been separated from his three hens for the whole of the night this wonderfully white Pekin drake couldn't wait to do his stuff.

'Does he always pick on the same hen?'

'Yes,' the young girl replied, 'it's always Apricot.'

And as sure as drakes are drakes, Apricot it was. The hens were just your standard sort of white laying pullets, bred principally to produce eggs and not go ten or fifteen rounds of Greco-Roman wrestling with a marauding drake. He grabbed the poor fowl by the throat and, jamming her head into the ground, proceeded to drag her all over the yard and then climb all over her for good measure. I had to pull out a referee's badge to break up the commotion.

It always needs a bit of an overview to sort out a solution. The back yard was a mirror image of the front, plus or minus the heaps of broken bricks. The young lass was keen to point out the better features of the chook pen, 'over here we installed a bath yesterday,' and sure enough, they had. Someone had gone to a whole lot of trouble to bury a full-size steel bath in the soil with the lip at ground level. 'It'll be great for the duck,' she said excitedly. I wasn't so excited.

'It's solution time!' advises Petrina.

'Right,' I thought. 'This is a doozey.'

'Baths buried like this are not a good idea,' I advised my incredulous young client. 'Ducks can't get out of them unless they are full to the top as the sides are too slippery, and they'll drown.'

'But our neighbour next door said ducks need water and so we put it in,' piped up Mother, who until now had kept right out of things. 'You'll have to forgive the place,' she added, 'we're renovating.' To anyone with even a semblance of knowledge about building, there was no obvious line here between renovation and demolition.

'Drakes are very assertive birds, he is the male picking on the lowest member of the chicken hierarchy, and attempting to display his dominance by mating with her.' They looked bewildered. 'Physical separation is the only answer. Keep the chickens in one pen, him in another and get a female for him, that will take away some of his bullying.'

There were a few mild protestations but basically the matter was agreed as I had suggested. Morning tea was served and the crew got stuck into the coffee and biscuits. With such an early start, hunger invariably sets in around mid-morning. Soon it was time to take our leave, more problems to solve, and hopefully no more drakes for a while.

'By the way,' I advised as we stepped over the threshold, 'watch that bath, because chickens can't swim, and ducks really love to mate in water.'

Safely in the car and out of earshot, we all had a bit of a chuckle. Surprising how many people don't realise that just because all birds have got feathers they don't all act the same. Petrina was rabbiting on about the next house call and where we should go for a decent lunch.

'You didn't have any coffee,' she asked, 'weren't you hungry?'

'No, I was pretty worried about the cockies.'

'What are you talking about, Harry, there were no cockies. They were chooks and a duck!'

'Not the sort of cocky you're thinking of. It was the big fat brown ones lying legs up all the way down the main hallway of the house that worried me, I counted seven or eight!' She wasn't ill, but she didn't enjoy lunch, that I can tell you.

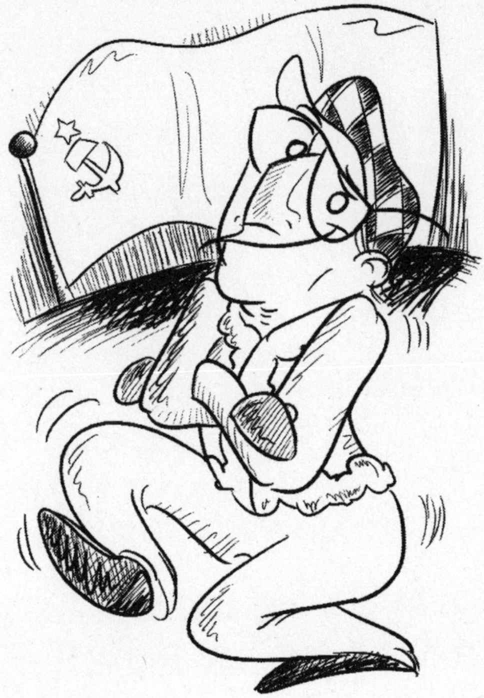

A Visit to Russia

22

Via Japan

My interest in birds really began with those first few budgerigars, given to me by my father before I started high school . . . with time a specialist knowledge developed, more through practical experience and observation than through book education. In those times there were very few vets interested in cage birds and even fewer books on the subject. In simple terms there was no one to teach it. With some application of scientific principles, a few of us had managed to gather together the very beginnings of knowledge on the subject. This led me to be invited to speak at the World Veterinary Conference.

Now this isn't something that happens every day of the week. These meetings are pretty major affairs and this one was going to be something special, because the venue was Moscow.

The subject of my presentation was simply 'bald cockies'. I hastened to explain to most of my colleagues in routine small animal practice, that this didn't mean ageing sheep farmers wearing large-brimmed hats to protect their shiny domes but rather a very specific disease of sulphur-crested cockatoos and other large Australian parrots. Back in about 1979, we did not know a heck of a lot about the problem but with the help of Professor Howlett, a fellow vet now teaching at university, and a few of my friendly pathologists we had managed to make some inroads into the possible cause of the problem. It would be many years later before the disease would be properly classified by veterinarians as being caused by a specific virus. We had a lot of clues back then but we didn't have the proof.

The temptation of such a journey induced a few of my colleagues to join the pilgrimage. The trip was planned with all the detail imaginable. You don't go to Russia every day of the week, do you? So when you do go, you want to have a damn good time and that was the object of the exercise. Somehow, like so many of today's 'business trips', the conference was the excuse for being there. The itinerary was complex. Initially we would all fly to Japan, and spend three or four days there exploring not only Tokyo itself, but the countryside as well. Then it would be on to the Russian east coast where the Trans-Siberian railway would be waiting. After three days' travel we would be halfway across. The plan was to get off, fly south, and spend a week or so checking out all the little provinces bordering Afghanistan. Even their names conjured up visions of the silk trade and exotic myths. Finally everyone would fly back to Moscow for the conference. It would take a little over fourteen days to reach our final destination. Some of the things that happened on the way are certainly worth recording.

The touring party comprised five couples altogether and we assembled as a unit for the first time in Tokyo. All the blokes were vets. First there was Greg, from around Turramurra way on Sydney's north shore, and his wife, a physio. Henry had a nice little practice down near Warriewood, close to the northern beaches. He brought along his wife Tania. Tim had a small animal practice on the lower north shore and his better half came as well. Dick, on the other hand, held down a government job in Canberra and his wife was a teacher, if memory serves me correctly. Lastly there was yours truly and my first wife, a pharmacist. Quite an interesting and diverse group, and luckily we all got along.

The two of us had left a few days earlier to spend a little time in Hong Kong. It was a truly fascinating place. Just so alive, and so friendly. All the tourist things like the Peak railway, the floating restaurants, the markets and Aberdeen were visited and enjoyed. You could never be bored in Hong Kong, and it was to set the mood for the rest of the journey.

If you've never stayed in a Japanese hotel then you've never learnt to live in a shoebox. It was our first experience of it, and, boy, if you suffered from claustrophobia you'd have been hospitalised within twenty minutes. Everything was in miniature, from the very room itself, to the bed, the dressing table, the wardrobes, even the teacups and teapot. The windows were more like portholes. You wouldn't want to spend too long in a joint like this, you'd go stir-crazy. Even back in the late 1970s everything you bought to eat, with the exception of noodles, put a severe dent in the old credit card. Japan is a very expensive country to visit.

Tokyo was enormous and the city itself was absolutely teeming with people. The public transport system functioned as you would expect of anything in modern-day Japan, like a well-oiled machine. To get from A to B was easy, you just got on a train. That was easy, too, because there were people there to make sure you did! Stand anywhere near a carriage doorway and you were certain to be shoved on by guys dressed in blue uniforms. These fellas had certainly been spending most of their spare time at the local gym, and by the look of their biceps perhaps had been swigging the odd anabolic steroid or two. Sardines on toast for brekkie is one of my favourites, and the suppliers have a habit of packing as many fish into a tin as possible. That's just the way a Japanese train functions too. It's hard enough to breathe, let alone maintain your balance. The one saving grace is that the trains travel at incredible speed, you reach the destination very quickly, and you can get out the door before feeling totally overcome. There is one proviso. You need to be standing very close to the door, because most of the people want to get on before you have a chance to get off. It didn't take too long to learn that if you wanted to get anywhere, you went into front row footballer mode and just shoved! After all, that's exactly what the locals did. To the system's great credit, everything was almost surgically clean. No lolly papers, cigarettes or refuse of any kind littered the platforms and everything functioned just so efficiently.

After only a day or so in the big smoke it was time to head out into the country. Once again we travelled by train, but this one was more of an intercity express than anything else. We had seats, they were pre-booked so no one else could grab them. Japan is a 'first in, best dressed' society. Once again the effectiveness of the whole transport system was incredible. The train left on time, and stayed on time for the whole journey. Everyone except for myself seemed to enjoy the trip immensely. I've got to confess that for me it was a little uncomfortable.

I'm a man who really enjoys his meat rare. I'd always wanted to sample steak tartare. This has to be the ultimate in rare meat. It's raw! There it was on the menu in our swanky hotel, mind you, every hotel in Tokyo is swanky. It just had to be ordered, didn't it? To this very day I'm certain that it's what they did to the meat that caused the problem, not the meat itself. Out came the waiter dressed in a really spiffy outfit carrying this round lump of raw mince on a huge plate. He placed the dish on the table, just fractionally out of reach. For some very good reason, he hadn't finished. Up comes this trolley, which must have had at least a dozen assorted bottles stashed at each end. He throws the meat on the trolley, starts kneading and pounding the lump with gloved hands, a dash of this, a shake of that, a dollop of the brown stuff, more of the white stuff, a few chopped bits; the damn thing's grown to twice its original size. Couple of raw eggs, couldn't be any more, surely, it's been twenty minutes he's been working this lump of meat over. Perhaps he's trying to restore it back to life! Or are we watching an embalming ceremony? The best was yet to come. This guy's a brickie too! Out comes the trowel. Sorry, he's not a brickie, he's a sculptor. Carefully and deliberately he coaxes this now enormous lump of somewhat tarnished meat into the shape of a heart. Why in God's name a heart? I wouldn't know. After nearly half an hour of sculpting and poking, kneading and pushing, there it is, on the plate in front of me. The lump didn't even look like raw meat now. It tasted fantastic with some fresh bread and a few greens.

It's obvious that even hardened Australian intestines somehow quake at the thought of a thousand herbs and spices. I say again, it wasn't the meat itself that was the culprit, but halfway along what should've been a delightful country journey the herbs and spices went into overdrive and so did the colon. Now an attack of the runs is something most Aussies can deal with when on holidays. You come prepared (particularly when you are a vet). There are tablets available to treat just about everything that can go wrong on a holiday overseas. The problem is, that the problem strikes with a whoosh and that is definitely the right word.

Have you seen a Japanese toilet? They look more like a

hand basin. There's no seat – well, certainly not on the railway model. You open the door and there staring at you from the floor is a huge ceramic shower base. It's set right into the floor with a fairly large central drain hole, for obvious reasons, and two sort of corrugated bits on either side. It's pretty shallow but then it's fairly enormous in surface area. The idea is to squat. Get both feet firmly planted on the rough bits. One on either side and then simply – well, I think you know what I mean.

This is fine and works well in a hotel, a restaurant or on a slow-moving ferry, but on a bullet train at something like 120 kilometres an hour it's a trifle more difficult. The track we were travelling on had lots of bends. You find yourself listing to the left and back to the right, praying only that the carriage will right itself at the moment of imminent release . . . Otherwise you may end up with a shoe-full!

Regrettably the first 25 per cent of the journey was spent surveying the inside of the bullet train's water closet. But that was the one and only tummy upset of the entire trip.

We were very fortunate on the trip. Greg spoke fluent Japanese and it was his detailed planning that led to the excursion being such a success. His knowledge of the country was such because he acted as a courier for a Sydney-based tour company. He was able to converse with the locals at every opportunity to such a degree that we ended up sharing the compartment with a charming young lady who had recently been voted Miss Isawakamatzu. She was like a pretty little doll, every detail of her make-up and clothing was exquisite. She relished the opportunity to improve her English while teaching us fundamental Japanese.

Even in those days there was always something disguising my polished dome. Back then it was an Akubra. Very few of the locals had ever seen anything like it and at every station stop we'd go into this ridiculous 'What's under my hat?' routine. It went something like this: train pulls up, huge crowd gathers around window staring and pointing at the only non-Japanese train passengers they'd ever witnessed. Gestures are made to lift the hat from its repose on my head. All are ignored. Suddenly there's a twitch, I feign a worried look, and a careful lifting of one corner of the hat, followed by a sneaking of thumb and finger underneath the brim and a grabbing of the imaginary thing that I've found under my hat. Then commences a pantomine examination by myself and all other occupants of our compartment of this 'thing' now held between thumb and finger. Without warning the thing escapes and jumps onto someone else – and so it went on at every railway station. It passed the time and amused the onlookers, it's the sort of ridiculous game you invent when the journey is a long one.

Our destination was a small resort hotel set way up in the mountains of the Japanese countryside. Greg chose well, it truly was a wonderful spot. In the winter it served as a ski lodge and holiday haven, and in the summertime as a retreat from the workaday world and a chance to luxuriate in the warm mineral springs which the hotel had been built around.

Everything inside was polished timber and glass and everywhere the staff were bowing and scraping. Boy, they could teach a few things to the average Aussie pub. Everybody wanted to help, from carrying luggage, to almost carrying you as well. Unpacking your cases, hanging clothes in the tiny wardrobes, and placing slippers by the door were all part of the service. Hang on a minute. 'Where's the bed?' The housemaid didn't understand a word of English, but then again, it is their country.

'Greg, old son, where do we sleep?'

'On the floor, mate.'

'The floor looks a bit bloody hard to me!'

'Don't worry, they'll sort things out, first thing we need is a bath.' No showers in this place, just baths and they are big ones. They're made out of rock, or rather carved into the rock. If you're a bit shy about getting your gear off in front of someone else, well, you're gonna have to stay dirty. One for the girls and one for the boys? Not likely, this is Japan. All in together. The water from the mineral springs on the mountainside was both warm and relaxing. Firstly there's a good soak in here, followed by a wash in the pool next door, then back in for another soak and you're ready for dinner. You feel fantastic, really invigorated!

Noodles, noodles and more noodles. You get used to it and eventually you even like it, it's the sauces and flavourings that make the meal taste good, and they are subtle and sometimes spicy. Now, where is that bed?

Can you imagine a polished timber floor, a mattress approximately half an inch thick and a pillow which is actually a rather oblique timber wedge not much bigger than the palms of two hands? That was it. Sleep well. Gee, next morning there was a bruise the size of a dinner plate on my right hip – oh well, you've gotta live like the locals. The funniest thing was watching the girls applying their makeup before breakfast. The mirror was as big as your standard snapshot photo and the dressing table like something out of a doll's house. There was no shelf to stand it all on, the contraption had to stay on the floor. So all five of the girls either squatted or lay flat out on their abdomen to make themselves beautiful for the day.

Everywhere you looked was green tea: pots, cups, more

pots, more cups, you only had to turn around and there'd be a cup of green tea in your hand. After my experience on the bullet train, and Greg's advice about the effects of the stuff, green tea consumption was kept to a minimum.

Having breakfast was one of the greatest sensations ever imaginable. The room was a huge glass atrium with views out to the surrounding countryside and woodlands. The mountains beyond were cloaked in a faint grey shroud of fairy floss as the clouds seemed unable to drag themselves away from the towering peaks. The sun streamed in fingers between the trees, and played upon the tables like hands on a keyboard. From strategically placed speakers the sound of birdsong echoed across the room from end to end. If there were ever a contest for atmosphere this place would win it hands down. Breakfast came on a big dark green tray divided into perhaps twenty portions, each one with its own little morsel of Japanese cuisine. Seaweeds, fish, vegies and a big bowl of soup. This was the real Japanese experience, this was the way they did it, not like some fancy inner-city hotel. We visited a Shinto shrine, met with a sumo wrestler, what else is left? It would be great to go back one day. As we departed all the staff lined up in a row, from the housemaids right up to the manager, all bowing as we walked along the line shaking hands and making farewells. Finally we all crammed into the taxis and away we went to the station and then the airport. Next stop, Vladivostok in the USSR.

23

Ah! Those Russians

Stepping off our Japanese airliner it was with some trepidation and a fair buzz of adrenalin that the party sallied forth for our first encounter with the Russian bureaucracy. Customs and immigration were a breeze, they actually seemed happy to see us. Visas and all that sort of stuff had, of course, been organised back in good old Oz.

Everything being in order, the ever-present guide took over. The one thing you learn right from the time you set foot on Russian soil is the impossibility of going anywhere or doing anything without the presence of a guide. These men and women are inscrutable, well-dressed, well-spoken and well-mannered Russians whose job it is to ensure that we poor simple westerners get to see the very best side of Russian life. Back in those days the Berlin Wall and the Cold War were very much a part of life. But this party was on 'official business'. After all, we were delegates representing our country at the upcoming veterinary conference. The fact that we were also tourists was immaterial to these guys.

The bus trip from the airport had been a well-rehearsed lecture on the do's and don'ts for visitors and the superb successes and accomplishments of the Soviet Union since the death of that poor old bearded gentleman, Lenin . . . no relation to John! Along the asphalt roadway our relatively luxurious bus passed every form of transportation, including a donkey cart, with the ageing animal only a year or two younger than the whiskery-faced old driver. The whole dilapidated contraption teetered along on equally ageing wooden wheels, every bit of it crying out for a coat of paint. There were pushbikes by the hundred, all pretty much of the same design, all in need of a good overhaul, and all equally devoid of any form of bright paintwork. The riders all had two things in common; a dour expression fixed on their faces and a heavy, coarse grey woollen overcoat to keep out the chill. Occasionally a luxury limousine with the official flag fluttering gaily from the bonnet would roar past, and there were certainly privately owned motor vehicles as well. All the makes and models were foreign to us. They were obviously a local product and only came in one or two designs, with a colour range of black, grey or navy blue. Public transport seemed to be mainly buses, all diesel powered, all chugging along and misfiring pathetically, while belching copious quantities of grey acrid smoke. Mind you, not every one of them was on the go, a good many were pulled up on the kerbside, where a throng of interested would-be mechanics were busy investigating the cause of an obvious engineering failure. Quite a number were totally abandoned, these must have been beyond repair, we concluded. The colour scheme of just about everything was either grey, black, dark blue, or violent red. Was everyone here colour blind? Petrol was cheap, diesel was cheaper (our guide told us so – they have plenty of the black stuff bubbling up from below ground), and repairs must have been cheaper still. Our 'superior class' conveyance was more like your average Aussie school bus, but it got there!

Our hotel was about two stars by Australian standards, but that's probably what we'd all expected. The rooms were quite large, but very sparsely furnished. There was only one word for the decor: drab. The windows were filthy, covered with a layer of grime that must have taken years to accumulate, interspaced with streaky patches where rain dripping from the gutter above had managed to erase a little of the sludge. You couldn't see very much through this mess, and what was visible appeared to be on the verge of collapse.

What a sensation the bathroom was. The tap handles came off in your hand. The rail in the bedroom wardrobe could hold no more than two shirts, before it came crashing to the floor. The doorknob fell off when the porter closed the door. The bedsheets were torn in places and the pillows smelt heavily of cigarette smoke. Russian cigarette smoke, so much more pungent than our Aussie brew.

Downstairs, dinner was a well-catered affair. In a large room and at one table, we foreigners were the centre of attention, not only from the waitressing staff, but from the locals too. The meal was plain, but nutritious and at least it was hot. Now, I'll bet you think everybody in Russia eats borscht, the famous beetroot soup. Well, you'd be wrong. Everyone had been warned this was the staple Soviet diet, but not a trace graced our table that night. The locals eat lots of different things, plenty of root vegetables and stacks of stews. All warm and hearty. Well, blow me down, they're just like us. Meals are plain, no fancy sauces here, mate, just a big lump of whatever vegetable it might be splattered on the plate and whatever meat that happens to be on the cheap list lobs alongside it. Spuds, cabbage, carrots and onions seemed to dominate the menu. Now we come to the good part. All this was washed down with a bottle or two of fairly reasonable local wine. Some of the beer was good, some of the beer was bad – but not that bad that you wouldn't drink it, I've yet to find any that bad. While the meals were part of the package deal we'd negotiated for the trip, the drinks were not included, but no matter, in the late 1970s the Aussie dollar was worth real money and even the wine was affordable. Let's face it, after a couple of days in Japan anything would seem cheap!

Down the hallway from the dining area the locals were gathering. We followed the crowd to the source of the noise and the bright lights. A disco! Unbelievable, a disco in Russia. One should always have an open mind when journeying around the world. Everyone outside the Iron Curtain thought these guys were so staid that if it wasn't written by Tchaikovsky it was anti-communist. Our re-education took less than a minute, just the time it took to recognise the music. What a shock! A DJ, seated behind a console with a pile of records and people dressed in something other than black, dancing the night away, determined to enjoy themselves. A little bit of colour and a few strobe lights served to illuminate the display being put on by quite a number of fairly inebriated forms gyrating around the floor. Guess what they're playing? Boney M, no less! You wouldn't believe it, first up on the turntable he's spinning 'Rah, rah, Rasputin'! must be a time warp, how could they play this stuff, let alone play it in Russia, when it's about a Russian? We would all find out over the next weeks that many things had changed, and that life for the young city dwellers was at least becoming enjoyable.

24

Have Samovar, Will Travel

The Trans-Siberian railway was an experience never to be forgotten. If you get the chance, do it, it really is one of the great train journeys of the world. When leaving from the east coast near Vladivostok, it travels northwards, skirting China before making a massive left turn and heading clear across what was then the Soviet Union to Moscow. Australia is a big country, but the USSR was enormous. The trip was to prove quite comfortable, and for once the mandatory guide actually deserted us and the whole group was left to its own devices.

It's a very large train in anyone's language. At the business end were two massive grimy diesel locos, and stretching back behind were a dozen or more carriages. Like so many of the buildings, the outside of the train looked pathetic. Inside, it was actually quite warm and cosy. The compartments were certainly spacious. The seating was leather, though its condition had suffered from the ravages of time. The remainder was either timber or cast iron, certainly cleaner than the outside, but tired, nevertheless.

Once on board we settled in quickly. Each couple had their own compartment, comprising a set of fairly wide double-bunks fixed at right angles to the direction of the train. There was a large table and comfortable bench to sit on during the day and a huge window through which to view the rolling countryside. (We made a point of cleaning our window at our first opportunity.) You may have heard of *The Never-ending Story*, and that was certainly how it seemed. The landscape just went on and on and on, for three consecutive days the train almost never stopped but passed along the way a constant stream of locomotives heading in the opposite direction, hauling their cargo of crude oil or timber. You would lose count, the number was incredible. We'd pass a train nearly every twenty minutes, some with well over thirty-five freight-laden carriages in tow. Strangely enough, there was virtually nothing in the way of passenger trains travelling in the opposite direction.

The countryside that the train travels through is just so expansive. So much of the landscape is covered by hundreds and hundreds, no thousands and thousands, of acres of timber. Birch, larch and other varieties of conifer disappeared over the horizon and into the spring sunshine. The resources such huge forests contained were immeasurable. How could they ever run out of such a seemingly inexhaustible supply of hardware? While there were no oilfields visible from the train, the evidence of yet another of nature's bounties could be seen in the thousands of rail tankers heading towards the east like juggernauts.

Early on there were plenty of villages, but as time and distance unfolded these became fewer and smaller. Most were built right alongside the railway tracks. The majority were a collection of fairly simple little dwellings, many looked to be made of mud brick, others were probably rendered brick or concrete; few were painted. All were small by Australian standards, most about the size of a three-car garage, with little windows and big chimneys belching thick white smoke. Properties seemed to merge one with another. There was no such thing as a boundary fence. In stark contrast to our dwellings there was no semblance of a garden, the villages had an air of dustiness and dryness. Cars were rare out here, in their place were donkey carts and bicycles – or people just walked. Waving out the window always brought an instant response, especially from the kids, who, like children the world over, were happy inventing their own games and playing them with youthful enthusiasm.

On every street corner stood a huge pole, not so much to support any electrical wiring or telephonic communication, but rather to hold up the thousands of loudspeakers. Huge, ancient-looking devices they were, like something out of the Great War, pointing to every direction of the compass. This was the propaganda machine in full swing. I doubt they had any radio or television back in those days. Music of the pretty heavy classical type interspersed with what sounded like a diatribe in the local tongue blared forth intermittently from these prehistoric megaphones. Skinny dogs raced up and down the streets, with the children clad in pretty simple coarsely woven clothing in hot pursuit. Strangely enough, everyone seemed irrepressibly happy, smiling and waving as we hurtled past.

On occasions the train would be forced to slow for the odd level crossing, and we'd catch sight of an ancient blue and cream diesel-powered commuter bus, laden down with luggage on top and with passengers almost hanging out of the windows. It was an insight into how the rural communities really lived. A daily stop was a great chance to get out and stretch the legs and, boy, did the locals make the most of these stops. Mind you, there wasn't a station, they just didn't have them, no platform, no siding, nothing like that. The train just stopped to take on water and fuel and provisions for the rest of the journey. Everybody clambered down the steep steps and onto the ground right alongside the tracks. The locals were obviously used to these stops and it was like the local Sunday market in the mall car park. You could buy anything – well, anything Russian, of course – and that wasn't much. Homemade biscuits we soon found to be the best value both in terms of taste and rouble currency. They were something like an Anzac bikkie and tasted great. Bottles of the local cordial were pretty vile, after the first sip it was 'no thanks' to all of these. Toys aplenty, but almost always the same thing on offer, they were wooden dolls and almost invariably babushka dolls. It makes you think, so little variety even in the toys for their children, but then these were simple people and they would jabber away to us as if we were fully conversant with the local lingo.

Every character you would wish to meet was there; wonderful old ladies with time etched so indelibly on their complexion and their hands. A smile almost perpetually on their faces, usually exposing an oral cavity in need of a fair degree of dental remodification and replacement. They would badger us from the time we got off till the time came to reboard, and it was more sympathy than anything else that forced a surrender – eventually you'd be persuaded to purchase something. Well, at least you could eat it. A long hollow toot from the whistle and we all climbed back on board. A few piccies to remember them by and the express moves off again.

Very occasionally there would be a stop at a major centre. Here there was a proper station and platform. Passengers would get off, and new passengers would get on. You'll never guess who got into our carriage. About half the Russian weight-lifting team! These fellows were in for a real good time. A couple of them could speak a bit of English and needless to say all the girls thought they were pretty easy on the eye. Not only were they physically quite superb specimens, but they were good on the vodka as well. The remainder of the trip developed into something of a sightseeing contest. Nothing to do with the scenery but rather who could see the bottom of a bottle first. I'm joking, it wasn't that bad, but we did have a few good laughs over dinner and after it!

The tucker wasn't as bad as we'd been led to believe. Apart from breakfast it was mainly hearty stews, and lashings of soup, all served with the utmost deportment in the dining car of the train. Four days on the trip and still no borscht as yet! Frankfurts – or whatever the Russian equivalent of frankfurt is – seemed to find their way onto the plate of at least one meal a day. Fair dinkum, I thought these were the national food of Germany, not Russia.

What made the whole journey quite distinctive was the samovar. What's that, you ask? Aah, cripes, I thought everyone knew that. It's a Russian teapot; well, you know, sort of. At the back of the train, or rather at the back of each carriage lived a samovar and the cabin steward or stewardess (they seemed to swap about a fair bit). It was their job to keep the samovar alive and kicking. It was something so typically Russian I doubt you'd see one elsewhere. The device was a magnificent silver, or perhaps chrome-plated, urn, ornately decorated, engraved and polished with an elaborate lid and a delightful tap protruding from the front like a spout. What kept it hot I'm not sure, time erases some memories; probably it was a small fire kept burning day and night. The contents of the samovar never quite boiled, they stewed and so did the tea, that's what filled the darn thing. On a regular basis more leaves and more water were chucked in this enormous stew pot, as the passengers (ourselves included) siphoned off the steaming brackish liquid that passed for tea. This was Russia! It was Russian tea, thick, black and with a strong smoky flavour. With enough sugar it tasted passable, and it was always there and always hot. After three days the ten of us alighted from our 'clackety clack' home. The train continued to Moscow, but we were headed for our next Russian experience – the airport!

25

The USSR by Plane

The flight from Omsk in central Russia to Tashkent, the capital city of what is now the independent republic of Uzbekistan, was quite an undertaking and without the services of our trusty guide I'm sure the party never would have made it. P'raps that's what they want you to think. We were met once again by a well-spoken, neatly dressed young lady. There must have been thousands of these guides right throughout the length and breadth of the country just to look after tourists. Then followed the bus trip, the obligatory lecture, the propaganda and the luggage handling. Every stage was so well rehearsed, she must have done it a thousand times before.

The airport was an unspectacular edifice. The usual drab colour and unimaginative architecture, enlivened only by the swag of red flags and score of banners featuring various Russian patriots. Getting through the huge crowd in the airport building took some doing, but these guides obviously carry enormous authority because the crowd parted like the Red Sea as we advanced. The good lady up front was busy yelling instructions and threatening various officials with clenched fists. Somehow all ten of us seemed to jump the queue with consummate ease, and with tickets in hand we were shown to the waiting area.

Being a stranger in a foreign land is a sometimes eye-opening experience and in Russia our party was accorded all the pomp and ceremony of a political entourage. Our designated waiting area was upstairs, in a special room, with food even. 'Don't get too excited,' says Henry. There was just one type of biscuit and just one variety of soft drink. There's no need to go too far overboard, we're only Aussies. A window in the back wall offered a view over the entire terminal area below. 'Have a look at this, mate,' says Greg, and with that the whole group assembled around for a closer look. Below us was the human sea that we'd just navigated. There must have been not just hundreds, but thousands of people. They looked poor, they *were* poor, clutching simple possessions wrapped up in towels or blankets. Battered old suitcases, worn-out satchels, unshaven faces, toeless shoes, well-worn sandals, thick woollen coats with frayed elbows and cuffs, caps pulled firmly down to provide what little insulation could be found against the elements. Children crying, mothers yelling, everyone huddling together against the cold. It could have been a refugee camp, but it wasn't. They were all waiting for a seat on a plane. Some had animals, goats on tattered rope leads, chooks of every colour in homemade crates. It was a pitiful and yet somehow amazing scene of human patience and endurance. They just simply sat or lay propped up against one another or the wall. That blank look of loneliness on so many faces, the air thick with despair, but this was the life they had, they knew nothing else and they seemed resigned to the situation. Sitting, waiting for a plane. There were no seats. Just the floor!

Russian aircraft back then were the sort of 'Acme' copies of our local models. Remember the T-jets? They were those huge things that used to fly around Australia with their tails stuck right up on top of the tail fin and two or three massive motors not under the wing but down the back alongside the tail. They were shockingly noisy, probably that's why we don't see them any more. The Russians had thousands of them, there was only one airline, Aeroflot, if you didn't go with that you didn't go at all. The problem with these Soviet aircraft was that when they copied the original they didn't get everything quite right. The Ruskies made one fundamental blue. They failed to get the centre of gravity in the correct place. As honoured guests we were expected to get on first; 'expected' may not be the right word, 'made', I think is more like it. There the ten of us were, all seated in the front rows of the aircraft, even the interiors of which seemed to have a remarkable resemblance to our own local makes and models. Seats were comfortable, aisles were carpeted. You got on, not at the front as usual but sort of in the middle of the fuselage, and no one else was allowed to board the aircraft until our party was seated. By golly, how good it is to be this important! Wrong again.

Henry's wife, Tania, proved to be a great asset on the rest of the trip. She spoke fluent Russian, something not even our guide, spy or whatever else you'd like to call her, had the faintest clue about, as she farewelled us at the bottom of the steps. The idea we were being treated so regally was soon to be shattered.

'Listen, you guys,' Tania whispered, 'the only reason we get to board first is because if they put passengers down the back to start with, the damn plane sits on its bum; the balance of this thing is so temperamental that nobody should sneeze until we get off the ground.' Funny, we all felt so much better after this revelation, I don't think. Behind us the remaining passengers began to board. Goats and sheep were bleating, chooks were crowing, the aisles were chock-a-block full of household paraphernalia and livestock. People were arguing over seats, an all-in brawl erupted between three passengers, this was unbelievable stuff. Eventually we got underway and off the ground. The pilots had all been militarily trained, I'm sure. The way they flew those passenger jets wasn't like anything we'd experienced anywhere else in the world. Mind you, the airport runway didn't exactly fill us with confidence either. At each end they'd parked a huge D9 bulldozer and on the apron alongside this contraption were the remnants of several aircraft that obviously didn't make it off the ground or joined the ground at far too rapid a pace for their own good. Will we be next? Hope not!

Take-off is something akin to what a crash-test dummy must experience in a seatbelt experiment. At the end of the runway the brakes are applied, the engines are then revved to well past the red line on the taco, I'm sure, and the plane explodes down the airstrip like Donald Campbell's *Bluebird* once the constraints are released. Then there's the climb. The ascent is something akin to vertical.

'If he doesn't level this thing out in a minute, we'll be in outer space,' says Greg. The plane just keeps going up and up. It's nigh on impossible to lean forward, the G-forces are pinning each one of us to our seats. You can't hear any soothing music playing. That's because there isn't any. The air-conditioning doesn't get too cold. There isn't any of that either. Instead it's so damn hot the condensation rolls down the windows and the inside lining. The interior of the aircraft looks like a tropical storm. We are ten minutes into the first of many legs that make up our journey, and all of us are having second thoughts about getting on another plane. Hang on, we're not down yet. Too right; then there's the landing.

This pilot seemed to make an approach to the airstrip more consistent with a strafing run on an unspecified target than any landing technique I'd witnessed before. The plane dived from some incredible height, again in an almost vertical plunge towards the earth before levelling out, feet above the tarmac, and landing with an incredible thud on what surely felt like square wheels. There was a look around the faces of the group which said, 'Thank God we made it', but no one was game to speak.

Alighting in Tashkent was like entering another world; well, almost, there was yet another guide to greet us! This time it was a male. Driving to the hotel was so different to driving in the bigger cities of the USSR. Sure the streets were wide and long, but the level of traffic was only a trickle. The accommodation was pretty much the same, though, nothing worked. The lifts, the staff, the shower, even the toilet were continually on the blink, and all of this when the Olympics were something like twelve months away.

It was the city and surrounds we'd come to see. So different from anything we'd all imagined. Turkey was about the only place I'd seen that looked anything like what lay in front of us. Afghanistan was very close by and the influences of its religion and cultural practices were all around. How different to the cities and towns we'd passed on the Trans-Siberian trip. Up there it is so cold that in places the earth never, ever thaws out completely. It's called the permafrost zone. Anything more than about forty-five centimetres below the surface of the ground remains permanently frozen. Here, in total contrast, it was dry, dusty and sandy. The temperature was vastly different also: really hot, just like back home. Except for the city's parks and gardens there was hardly a blade of grass to be seen. In short it was all but desert. The domes, minarets and pointed arches of Islamic architecture dominated the city skyline, interspersed between modern blocks of high-rise accommodation. The people, too, were so different. Their dress was almost Arabic, and the colour, how good it was to see colour in clothing after the drab, lacklustre clothing of the north. Gone too was the green of the trees and the huge expanses of agricultural land. Gone the grey buildings and grey people. In their place everything a soft but somehow dirty cream, yellow, orange and perhaps even white. Cripes! Nearly forgot one thing, red flags, red flags, red flags, pictures of Lenin, more red flags. These were big; not your standard sort of political photo at voting time, they were gargantuan. Some two or three storeys high and half a building wide! We were beginning to feel at home again already.

Tashkent for a day and then on to Samarkand, where there were more of the same fascinating places – temples, ornately decorated with spires and domes, and chips of bright blue – began to appear. The odd entranceway still showed remnants of the original gold leaf which adorned it in a former time. Sad to see once-beautiful temples now so seemingly poor and devoid of even the most basic convenience that we would take for granted.

Bargaining became rather entertaining, it was without a doubt the only way to shop. The local populace really craved so many of our western niceties. Biros, for instance. Biros were worth a fortune, they sold for the Russian equivalent of about five dollars each. Stockings, boy, did the girls do a roaring trade with stockings, you could get a good bottle of vodka for a pair of stockings, I kid you not. And we had come very well prepared with plenty of contraband to offer!

Russian toilet tissue is sold in Australia by most hardware

stores. There is, however, a difference in name, back here it's black and goes under the heading of wet and dry sandpaper. Sure the Russian stuff was a dirty shade of cream, came on rolls and hung on the wall just as any toilet tissue does, but it had two sides (come to think of it, doesn't everything?). One side was for burnishing, the other for polishing. Neither was for wiping. We out here in the land of sunshine are really spoilt with our double-layered, super-soft, embossed, daren't-scratch-your-bum toilet tissue. According to one company even the ducks use it and if you've ever had to clean up duck manure, then you know it has to be good. Well, over in Russia it sure was thick, it was tough and it was all-but water repellent. If you had a roll of it and an industrial sewing machine, you could probably turn it into a waterproof coat. To say it was non-abSorbent (sorry about the pun) would be a monstrous understatement. But the group was ready for this too and a roll of the old Aussie Sorbent was worth one good bottle of Bulgarian champagne!

The toilet seats were something else as well. Many of them were made from compressed timber, which is pretty good except when the showerhead directs a fair percentage of its flow at the said toilet seat. Chipboard and water don't mix; well, they do but something has to give. So when seated on this particular throne one must spend some considerable time removing splinters from the circular imprint left on both cheeks.

The hotel bathroom was a ripper, too. The floor drain and the shower drain were both at the highest point of the floor. Only after fifteen centimetres of water had accumulated in the recess would it start to drain away.

At 2.00 a.m. that morning, the whole floor was woken by a crashing thud. Tim's mirror had fallen right off the front of his wardrobe and landed with a loud explosion on the floor as slivered glass radiated to every corner of the room. There were staff and uniformed officials crawling all over the place, sweeping and cleaning. What a shemozzle. Tim underwent a detailed cross-examination by the touring party the next morning, but swears to this very day that there were no high jinks going on. 'The damn thing just fell off while we were both sound asleep.' I believe him.

There was no need to worry about the guide not staying right alongside us while we slept. Her duties were taken over by another group of typically Russian workers. Russia is full of l.o.l.s, you find them everywhere. If you're not careful they bob up right beside you and the most predictable thing is that on every floor of your hotel you can find at least two of them. Generally speaking, you find l.o.l.s at either end of the hotel corridor, they're easy to pick, they're always dressed in black and usually knitting – and that's in black too. They never look up, but they know and see all that happens in their particular jurisdiction. Inside each one of them is a counting machine. You are counted in, you are counted out and if you are missing, look out! What concerned us all was simply this: with the massive concentration of l.o.l.s in every hotel in which we'd stayed, would there be enough for Moscow in the months ahead? What's an l.o.l.? Everyone's got them, but the Ruskies invented them and then patented them. A little old lady.

The flight from Samarkand to Yerevan was something else. The hour of departure was late, well after midnight. Once again our party was ensconced in the special area saved only for foreigners (who should have known better). Wending our way through the sea of people and animals in the departure lounge, stepping over goods and chattels, whilst dodging children, animals and people asleep on the floor en route to the departure gate. Escaping onto the tarmac is a relief from the oppressive atmosphere of the airport building, but it's frightening to look around and see a human tidal wave descending upon the exit lane. It was good to be on board as the usual gaggle of two- and four-legged passengers followed us up the gangway. Strangely enough, the door to the cockpit was open, and a fairly heated debate was in full swing. I will translate via Tania exactly what was said.

Pilot to engineer: 'What's this flashing orange light?'

Engineer to pilot: 'I don't know, I've never seen it before.'

Pilot to engineer: 'Don't you know what it means?'

Engineer to pilot: 'No, I don't, but if it's worrying you I'll turn it off.'

Pilot to engineer: 'Won't it just go off if everything is all right?'

Engineer to pilot: 'Everything *is* all right, except this orange light.'

Pilot to engineer: 'Well, I'm not taking off with this thing flashing.'

Engineer to pilot: 'I'll fix it, pass me the pliers.'

Pilot to engineer: 'What are you going to do with those?'

Engineer to pilot: 'Cut the damn wire!'

After a word-by-word translation of the quandary in the cockpit, do you think we were feeling nervous? We were. For fully five minutes these two argued about the importance of the flashing orange light. Thank heavens the pilot won. We all got off the plane, and stood as two separate groups, them and us, on the tarmac. The guide had long since departed and it was to be us versus the might of Aeroflot. We were last off, we had to be, or the aircraft would've sat on its bum. So, there the ten of us are, no guide, no nothing, just ten little Aussies standing on the airstrip at Samarkand. The pilot took charge, he couldn't speak a word of English, but any idiot can understand hand signals. He approached our group, struck a salute-like pose and pointed down the airstrip. We walked. We walked a long way. In all, around half a kilometre. Finally we came across a whole row of these 'Acme' T-jets. Then we all played that famous children's game, 'eeny, meeny, miney, mo, pick one plane and then we'll go'. At last a decision. This one looks good, we'll all get on this one. We did without argument, no flashing lights this time, and away we went. Fantastic! Yerevan and Tbilisi were to be our last stops before the conference in Moscow.

Some people take things literally. The whole lot of us had been in the USSR for something like ten days and not once had we feasted on the dreaded borscht. Every person we'd encountered before our departure had warned of a never-ending supply of the stuff. Where was it? A man could go into withdrawal. But one of our party was always prepared. Tim had read up on it. From detailed research he knew what Soviet food was all about. Our good friend Tim must have been a boy scout in his former life. This affable vet was prepared – well, about 95 per cent prepared – for any and every culinary emergency. Having arrived at Yerevan in the early morning with the sun only a pale imitation on the horizon, we filed down the gangway from our flight. We all had our feet firmly on the ground when Tim reached the bottom step. The poor man screamed in agony and collapsed on the tarmac. Blood gushed from his leg. 'Strike,' we all thought, 'he's cut himself on the gangway'. No such luck. No compo payouts for you,

Tim, not that you'd win if you sued the Ruskies, anyhow . . . let me explain. All this talk about borscht had gone right to Tim's head (obviously bypassing his stomach on the way). He and his good wife had both convinced themselves that a staple diet of this traditional dish would be akin to starvation or food poisoning, or perhaps both! No way were either of them gonna eat the stuff. He'd come well equipped with some good old Aussie tucker. Tinned ham. Now it's fine having tinned ham but you don't exactly eat it with a spoon. Nor do you push it into your mouth whole, like a diner at a medieval banquet. You cut it, neatly, into thin slices and for that, gentlemen, you need a knife. Tim had one: it was a thirty-five centimetre razor-sharp carving knife, which after ten days and heaven knows how many trips had managed to work its way through the end of his faithful Qantas carry bag (Aeroflot don't have them) and into the side of his thigh.

It was a massive gash, a good ten centimetres long and at least four centimetres deep. The blood was fairly pulsing out of the wound. Vets knew what to do, we applied a pressure bandage and literally threw him to the wolves, heavily disguised as the Russian medical profession. This good lady must have been the mother of one of those weight-lifters we'd met earlier on the train – she was just as big, and almost as hairy. She examined the wound with the callousness of a forensic pathologist, and prepared to close the gaping hole with some sutures. The stuff she was gonna stitch him up with I'd have used on a draughthorse. Still, with a little bit of help from us and somebody explaining to her in Russian what local anaesthetic was, Tim finally got sorted. By the time he'd finished his first-hand encounter with the Russian medical system, veterinary practice seemed a pretty good alternative.

The wound certainly held together all right: you could have anchored the *Queen Mary* in a North Sea gale with the suture material and the bandage was so thick that it could have doubled as a well-applied plaster cast. He declined the wheelchair. We assisted him to the waiting ambulance and thence to hospital.

The person most perplexed by Tim's plight was, of course, the guide. Who should he stick with – us or Tim? With us, naturally enough, and poor old Tim spent half the night in the local hospital's outpatients' department. He did look a pretty sorry sight the next morning at breakfast. But there were enough pain relievers on hand to cheer the poor lad up. Antibiotics for infection? He didn't get any. What were they? Luckily we had some and suggested that as sterility was only an intermittent visitor to the casualty room he'd better take them. This was the one event that even Tim wasn't prepared for.

26

Come On In, the Water's Fine

A major feature of so many cities we'd encountered was the seemingly interminable memorials and statues and civic buildings, they would have done our own public servants proud. There was a monument to this patriot and that patriot, to Lenin, of course, to people who died in various wars and the most important statues of all, those celebrating the workers. All had the same sort of theme: 'Come on, lads, let's get on with it' and they did, but in a pretty slow and leisurely fashion. Everything was so stark, no advertising, no billboards, no hoardings, no flashing lights – believe it or not, we started to miss them. Just red flags and the same mass-produced picture of good old Lenin. Even the flowerbeds were either red or white and there weren't too many of those anyhow. The people walked with heads bowed, never daring to look you in the face. At least here in Yerevan the clothing was lighter, not like the heavy garb of the northern areas.

For the girls the trip lacked one essential. There was nothing to buy. The shops all sold the same stuff. It was all made by the state, and it all looked the same. Take shoes, for example, you could have one of two styles in any size you liked as long as the shoe was black in colour.

But it was a lovely sunny day and exploring the city with our very congenial guide was quite good fun, even though after a time all the damn monuments began to look the same.

Yerevan is the capital city of what is now the republic of Armenia. It is very close to Turkey. 'What's the chance of a Turkish bath?' enquired Greg of the guide. He looked puzzled, and pretended not to understand. Obviously he didn't want to get involved. But Greg was a pretty persistent fella. He'd been asking this same question of every guide since we left the Trans-Siberian and at last this one seemed to have some sort of clue. Just that small insight was enough for Greg to drive in the wedge.

'Where do we go?' A shrug of the shoulders.

'You just show us, we'll do the rest.' More shrugging of shoulders.

'Go on,' and the flash of a US ten-dollar bill sealed the deal. A taxi from the hotel was organised.

'Who's coming?' asked our faithful leader. Henry and myself and our wives fronted up in the foyer. This was going to be something special.

Taxis are only allowed to carry four passengers; three in the back and one in the front. There were six of us. The girls lay on the floor in the back, reminiscent of those days at the old drive-ins. Detailed instructions were given to the driver by a somewhat concerned and at this stage fairly nervous guide and we were on our way.

The driver had obviously been taught how to handle a motor vehicle by Michael Schumacher. The taxi left the hotel entrance like a dragster burning off the starting grid, belching smoke from all tyres and squealing like a piglet in mortal distress. He threw the car from one side of the road to the other with some sort of maniacal frenzy. We ducked and dived and dodged and totally dismissed any hope of getting to the place alive. This guy was a fruit loop of the first order.

Grabbing hold of the wheel with his right hand he spent more than half the time turning round to the passengers in the back gibbering away the whole time in Russian. If the damn thing hadn't been on autopilot we'd never have made it. Dead-set, half the journey must've been on the wrong side of the road. Finally we arrived. Then there was the question of the fare. Roubles weren't worth too much and yet if there was enough of them then they really did add up, and you had to be a little careful flashing too many US dollar bills around the place, everyone was a spy. The state was the boss. I couldn't see any meter on the dash. He was gesticulating in hand signals, shoving one hand into a pocket, holding up fingers; God knows what he meant, I didn't. We all piled out of the back seat onto the kerb except for Greg, who from the front seat was now involved in a heated debate with the driver about the fare. Suddenly a woman appeared out of nowhere. She seemed to know the driver. They began arguing as well. She wanted Greg's jeans. Damn the money, get his trousers. The whole mess developed into a tug of war, us pulling him out of the car and them pulling his jeans in. A good pair of Levis, even a bad pair, was worth a lot of roubles. A crowd was gathering, things were looking a little nasty, then suddenly all went quiet. Some bloke in a uniform turns up. Threatens everyone with a gun. The crowd disperses and we retreat into the foyer of the bathhouse.

I think we won. Greg kept the jeans. 'Let's hope we don't get the same bloke on the way back,' says Henry. The building looked something like a mosque with all the towers and peculiar domed roofs that tapered to a point with a thin spire on top. The entranceway was an elaborate arch finished in the same architectural style as most of the local places of worship.

At last there was a bit of colour, some blue tiles struggled to glisten through the general grime of the establishment.

Once inside, the place stank, and I mean really stank. Something akin to a thousand rotting eggs. 'What are we doing in here?' said the girls almost in unison. But Greg was determined, this was a Turkish bath and like it or not we were all gonna have one. He fronted the counter. In reality it was more like a ticket window at an old-fashioned theatre, staffed by a swarthy-skinned, massively overweight gentleman in his mid-fifties. Sign language to the fore again? No. Score one for our guide, he'd actually thought ahead and ordered the whole thing. All we had to do was pay. Greg shoved under the window the note kindly written by our guide. It detailed the sort of treatment that we'd requested. Heaven knew what was involved but we were soon to find out.

Money changed hands, and the party was ushered inside. To the locals we must have looked so different. Their dark skin, somewhat oily olive complexions and jet black hair were completely the opposite of our own. The majority of the local male population had at least some form of facial hair, either goatee beards or thin moustaches, while the women had huge tresses of jet-black hair that hung halfway down their backs.

The steps from the entrance led immediately downwards and when we reached the second level the ladies were escorted to one side. We fellas went on down one more floor, to be greeted by an obviously recently retired member of the ubiquitous Russian weight-lifting team. Standing right in the middle of the passageway like a colossus with arms folded, he was not about to let us go anywhere. He smiled slowly, perhaps he knew what was in store for us poor westerners. Slowly and deliberately this keeper of the depths nodded his head up and down a time or two, and unfolding his huge hairy arms, pointed to a small room off to one side. Anyone with any brains at all could tell that this was the changing area and with appropriate sign language that's exactly what was indicated to the three of us. 'You go first, mate,' says Greg to me. There didn't seem to be much choice in the matter. The weight-lifter indicated in no uncertain fashion that I should in fact remove all remaining clothing, including the undies that still hid my modesty. Spectacles too, he indicated; they had to come off as well. Now I'm really in trouble, everything's a blur, well, pretty close to it. 'Shove your clothes in the locker,' he said in Russian. We did it anyhow, who was gunna argue with this bloke? He closed and secured each locker with a large bolt. Funnily enough, I didn't think anyone was about to knock our gear off anyhow, not with this bloke standing guard. He must have been six foot three!

His thick brown finger pointed down the corridor and with a flick of the wrist he indicated the direction I should travel. The other two were still fussing about with their clobber. Entering the room through a narrow doorway, I could see nothing special to suggest this was any sort of a men's bath club. The floors and walls were wet and smelly, there was a very stingy beam of light entering through a narrow shaft that ran to the street above. It even felt dark, and certainly more than a little steamy. At one end of this dank room a length of rusting pipe hung from the ceiling. From it sprouted three or four protrusions where showerheads used to be. Instead a yellow icicle of solidified sulphur hung in its place. Sulphur dioxide with a stench like rotting eggs filled the whole chamber. What do you do? There were no instructions written anywhere, not that I could have read them anyhow. So being the first in line, and rather than standing alone in the centre of the place, I thought it best to jump under a faucet and turn on the water. The smelly yellow soup began to trickle all over me. I've smelt better after ten days in the outback without a shower. Sure the stuff was hot, but if this was all there was then we were paying big money for very little!

Remember a movie character called 'Odd Job'? James Bond does. He tangled with this very resourceful Oriental individual in one particular classic. Imagine Odd Job multiplied to three times his size. That's about the stature of this bloke who spontaneously appears from an even darker doorway. He's the masseur, the bather, the torturer, or whatever else you'd like to call him. When he entered the room everyone shook except yours truly, who couldn't even see him. He was behind me. I was discontentedly trying to keep my body warm under the trickle from above, when suddenly a large hand made firm contact with my shoulder. A quick turn to the left, bloody hell, there he was! The same massive paw grasped my left arm and propelled me physically towards a concrete bench, in the diagonally opposite corner. There was some sort of indication, both verbal and otherwise, that I should get up on this slab. I was too slow. He got me up. In one breathtaking motion I was hoisted bodily from the floor and flung down on the wet concrete. Lying there flat out and face down on this slab of chilly sand and cement like some sacrifice on a prehistoric Druid altar, you naturally work your way as quickly as possible to the rear. Fat chance, two massive hands grabbing every spare inch of skin covering your back, pull you into the centre. Now I'm exactly where he wants me. Boy, does he want me. (The rest of the treatment I can only report second-hand, as told to me by Greg and Henry, who didn't need glasses to catch the action.)

Crash! A massive hand lands fair in the middle of the poor sufferer's back. Breathing instantly becomes impossible, I struggle to gasp just a little air. For certain, three lumbar vertebrae and two ribs have already been broken. Crash – down it comes again. This time there was a splattering of soap followed by rubbing and pounding. The sponge in his mitt was more like a lump of sandstone. The rubbing he'd perfected while working in a metal machinery shop. Every square centimetre of the rear part of the anatomy was eroded to a depth of at least two millimetres. He had exposed layers of skin that had never even seen daylight before. Protest was impossible; breathing was difficult enough. Thank God I couldn't see. 'If he does the same thing to the front half, I'm dead.' Praying the ordeal would soon be over. Bad use of the word.

'Over you go.'

'God, not again!' This time I actually see this huge hulk of a man soak his sponge in a wooden tub of sudsy water sitting alongside my pummelled frame. The other two are laughing themselves silly, I can barely make out their naked forms through the soap in my eyes. Their turn would come and they didn't have as much material as I did for him to work on. The sadist was no easier on the front of my anatomy than on the rear. Worse still, this time I could see him coming.

This must finish soon or there'll be nothing left to take back to Aussie. Finally, after fully ten minutes of this totally abrasive undertaking, what remained of my frail human form was hauled from the table, repositioned vertically and frog-marched towards the bath.

Trouble was, it wasn't a bath at all. A sort of miniature indoor swimming pool would be a better description. The structure was made from solid concrete, none of your fancy tiles or pebblecrete finishes on this one. This was raw Soviet construction at its purest. The thing was filled almost to the brim with fluid. No one in their right mind could call it water. Standing in this cesspit the liquid rose to a depth just below my armpits. It was black, it stank and it was warm with an almost supernatural sort of putrid mist rising from its surface like some massive witches' cauldron. Out of breath and out of skin, the whole body sank into this evil mess.

Up periscope! U-boat off the starboard bow! Look out, there were other blokes in there with me. All you could see were their little black moustaches and their eyes at water level. For certain the two of them were loaded with depth charges or some other horrible weapons. They were so black and I was so white. Like a standing start at the trots, we're off. First, a slow and deliberate walk around the outside of the pool, which, incidentally, was probably only three metres square. It didn't take long for the walk to speed to a canter and from the canter to a gallop, and, strike, a man couldn't find the steps to get out.

'Henry, Greg, where are ya? We need some reinforcements!!' The cavalry arrived, the U-boats left and we had a damn good laugh. As a matter of fact, it's the story that went on to become the highlight of the whole trip.

We three stagger up the stairs looking and feeling like we've just been to hell and back. The girls are waiting, they're all smiles and laughing. They've had a wonderful time with the locals. Tania, of course, could speak the lingo. No torture for them, just simply a mild wash and a thorough shampoo of their hair. The local ladies were fascinated by the different colours of the girls' hair and their styles too. For they wore their hair only one way, long and natural.

For many of the locals this torture was a regular weekly

experience. Quite honestly, though, it's an experience I'd prefer not to repeat, but in a way a fitting end to our tour of just some of the various cultures that, back then, made up the massive USSR.

27

The Main Event

Our last flight on this leg would be to Moscow. In many ways it was similar to the ones we'd had before. We get on the plane first. We hear the squabble from down the back, and pray the thing gets off the ground and down again without them having to scrape us up with a bulldozer. Unbeknown to us, Moscow had five airports. We also had no idea which one we were headed to, but the rest of the passengers did. Towards the end of the flight things started to get just a little bit restless down the rear of the plane.

'What's going on down there?' Henry asked Tania to try to translate.

'Well,' she said, 'it looks like we're off to the wrong airport. All the locals have bought their tickets for one particular destination. We are, apparently, heading for a totally different one.'

Trouble was brewing; the closer we got to our destination, the more agitated the passengers became. The poultry joined in the chorus of protest. Ducks were squabbling in the aisle, chickens were flapping and carrying on a treat. The turkeys grew more restless by the minute. That's not to mention the goats and the sheep, who by now were really getting quite stirred up.

'Geez,' said Greg, 'if the animals know we're heading to the wrong spot, what's the pilot up to?' People were jumping on seats and yelling abuse, throwing things, and altogether were thoroughly displeased with what was happening. Strike, we had no idea.

'Keep your heads down,' said Tim as missiles rained against the cockpit door. You are probably wondering what the cabin staff, you know, hosties and the like, were doing about all this. Welcome to domestic Aeroflot. There weren't any cabin crew!

Once the plane touched down, the pandemonium turned into a riot. Stuff was going everywhere. Passengers were hurling abuse and anything else they could find at the cockpit. Talk about being in the wrong place. The garbage was piling up around us as we crouched in our seats. I ask you, where is a guide when you need one? We'd never encountered anything like it so far on the trip. Halfway down the runway everything stopped. The plane. The engines. (Not the air-con, because it never really started.) He just parked it, slap-bang in the middle of the runway. The cockpit door flew open. There stood the captain, behind him the engineer. Tania translated.

'You are in Moscow. You wanted to be in Moscow, you are in Moscow!'

There was more uproar.

He drew a revolver from its holster, pointed it in the air, then at the locals.

'We are all in Moscow!' What more could he say?

Silence reigned, we were in Moscow, thanks very much. They all got off, not another murmur, not even from the animals.

We had a two-hour wait for the guide and the bus. Sorry, fellow passengers, this was not the airport the flight was due to land at. The pilot was wrong, but when you've got a revolver in your hand you're never really wrong, are you?

I suppose when staying in the country's capital we'd hoped for something just a little more upmarket. No such luck, here we are in the same sort of hotel, with the same never-ending supply of little old ladies, and the same crummy lifts. But you'll never guess what was on the menu for dinner that first night. You've got it in one – a huge bowl of borscht! Welcome to Moscow! There are many things about the city that drag you out of a boring hotel room and challenge you to look around. We'd arrived on a Saturday night. Sunday would be just the ideal day to go exploring.

From an architectural perspective so much of the past had been preserved. After all, Moscow had escaped the ravages of the Second World War, which had destroyed so much of neighbouring Europe. There were virtually no restrictions on our movements in the city. Walking is one of the best ways to get a proper feel for the place. The famous view from across the river, of the Kremlin and that stunning group of buildings with their cathedral steeples and shining domes and spires is every bit as good as it looks on television today. Red Square is huge, it's partly paved, and even in the quiet cold of a Russian morning, there are people about. Their dress is more ordered, they look a prouder people with perhaps a little more in their pockets than their country cousins have. Lenin's tomb is quite awe inspiring, standing as it does almost at the very centre-top of the square. There was always a stream of viewers. Somehow it's always the little things that stick in my memory.

Moscow is a very clean city, you could eat a meal right off the pavement without fear of contamination. On the other hand, much as I love the very life and atmosphere London exudes, it is probably the dirtiest joint I've ever seen. Why the difference between two such great cities? It's simple, every

Sunday that wonderful band of l.o.l.s trots out and washes the whole place down. No kidding, they just buckle up hoses to all the fire hydrants around the place and with high-pressure water, and plenty of it, they hose everything in sight and the lot disappears down the drain. Come Monday, Moscow comes up shining. There isn't a square centimetre that you couldn't use as a dinner plate, and as for the railway – well, the underground is quite fantastic.

London's 'Tube' is the envy of so many cities right around the globe, with its ongoing expansion of subterranean train travel on a multitude of different networks. But it is complicated. Ticketing is a nightmare for the inexperienced, there's much walking and travelling on escalators to get from one line to another, and to top it off it's pretty grubby. Moscow's 'Metro' would pick it up and carry it. No tickets, no lolly papers, no vending machines and no smoking – equals no mess. There is just nothing lying around or cluttering up the place anywhere! Passengers pay as they go through the barrier and once through, they can go anywhere on the system. One initial fixed charge covers the traveller anywhere, and you can get off and back on as often as you like, as long as you don't exit through the barriers. (Sounds like 'Charlie and the M.T.A.', the Kingston Trio song.) The stations are elaborate, every one is different. Some feature valuable works of art, others have their walls decorated by huge murals or frescoes. One was totally illuminated by stunning glass chandeliers, while the next one along the line displayed superb masonry and sculpture. Could you imagine how long this sort of thing would survive in the west; vandalism would ruin it in one night. Three or four hours spent riding on the system is a truly rewarding experience. Clocks advise how long ago the last train departed and how long till the next arrives. The trains themselves are state of the art and extremely comfortable, quiet and very spacious, mind you, this was a Sunday, and no one could tell us what it was like at peak hour on a workday. The whole system runs with the sort of efficiency you wish existed in our own railway systems.

Yet for all of this, for the magnificent splendour, and the extravagant wealth of the Czars on public display, the average citizen was certainly not all that well off. Women queued for hours for simple loaves of bread. Vodka was in short supply and could only be purchased with coupons. On many street corners stood ageing women selling simple items like books of matches and shoelaces from mobile stands that should have been condemned many eons ago. Every city has contrasts. The difference between wealth and poverty was here in Moscow for all to see as well.

The conference commenced on Monday and it was a real eye-opener. We had expected things to be a bit of a shambles. How wrong can you be? Delegate registration, the collection of documents and notes, our invitations to dinner and so on were all managed with ease and efficiency. The whole kitbag and caboodle was presented in a stiff blue plastic carrycase. Yours truly even scored a special badge, with a slash across it, being a guest speaker and all that. I, for one, was quite looking forward to the whole event.

A welcoming cocktail party was planned for the first night. Being pretty well the only Australians at the event we thought it best to attend as a group, moral support and all that sort of stuff. Very few others had made the trek.

It was a huge event; once again, as Aussies we really stood

out – talk about laid-back. Everyone else wore dark suits, with contrasting white shirts and equally sombre ties. (Not the ladies, just the blokes, but frankly the local female attendees didn't look much better – dull was in!) We're a blaze of colour. The ladies in their best gear shone in reds and yellows and browns. The fellas, not to be outdone, showed up complete with Akubras and the like. Real sunburnt country stuff. To commence there's plenty of mingling, though even Tania has trouble interpreting what some are saying, followed by polite sipping of wine, and the traditional skolling of vodka (no coupons needed), ending with a choking glass of the local cloudy beer.

The doors flew open to the banquet hall, and something akin to a tidal wave swept past us. It's not difficult to imagine what happened to the Mona and Eida dams when the dambusters dropped their deadly load. Yeah, the water surged through like an unstoppable avalanche. So it was with the delegates. Talk about pigs to the trough. By the time our group got in there was absolutely nothing left. People can at times behave like animals but perhaps that's doing our animal friends an injustice. To see adult human beings shoving food into their mouths with both hands, and into their pockets and handbags at the same time, defies belief. No one begrudges anyone a meal, but none of them looked as if they needed it anyway. They were not skinny, quite the reverse, the majority were obese. Now we know why they all dressed in black! Perhaps in hindsight they were going at the food like that because it was free, but in my eyes that will never excuse the behaviour. We ate not one thing, but went out, swapped another pair of pantyhose for a couple of good bottles of vodka and got room service. Well, that's what they called it!

The moment had finally arrived. The reason for my epic trip from Sydney to the World Veterinary Conference was now.

'Dr Harry Cooper from Australia will present his paper on feather loss in sulphur-crested cockatoos,' stammered the German chairman, in stilted English. 'Dr Cooper, you have seven minutes.'

Well, that's fine by you, old fella, it'll be closer to quarter of an hour by the time I've finished. I didn't travel halfway around the world to speak for just seven minutes! Besides the cheer squad was in the audience and I'd primed them with several questions to ask. Just as well they were, the topic wasn't a riveting one unless you were into birds, and nobody was, twenty-three years ago. My total audience probably numbered no more than twenty. A quick glance suggested that at least ten were sound asleep. Off came the Akubra and as there were no hooks on which it could hang, the best bet seemed to be the other microphone. Strike a light, this German chairman went right off his cruet. He's gesticulating and waving and carrying on and motioning me to remove it. Funny how you can't understand a word once you've got the podium. Ah, leave it there, I'll use this other microphone, I reckoned.

The talk was going well, we were halfway through my slide collection, when at six minutes, the buzzer rings. Funny, I couldn't seem to hear that either. At seven minutes the wretched buzzer has gone into overdrive, if he keeps his finger on that damn button it'll go into meltdown. I'd learnt a little from Tim about being prepared, and snuck in the day before to get the lie of the land. Directly underneath and slightly to the right on my lectern there's a switch. Flick it and bingo! That killed the power to the buzzer. The poor bloke after me was talking about some egg-laying problem in Arctic sturgeons, they make caviar, that's all I know. Who wants to hear about egg-bound fish, anyhow? Exactly twelve minutes into the talk my chairman has his face buried in both hands, his deputy is still pleading with me to finish. I take a question (well rehearsed, of course) from the floor, he realises that my subject is at least of interest to someone and allows the talk to continue. When you've got the stage . . . hold it . . . that's what my mum taught me, for that's where she grew up. The applause wasn't generous, but it was well meant. I picked up the Akubra, thanked the profusely sweating chairman and exited stage right.

Oh yeah, forgot to tell you, the special little slash on my badge was red, of course!

No trip to Russia would be complete without a visit to the circus and the ballet. Our Moscow guide was a very evasive lady. She would have made a good politician, no straight answers to any questions.

'Who would like to go to a ballet?' Hands go up.

'What sort of ballet?' Never mind what sort of ballet, I reckon we're in Russia and they're out to impress us, so it'll be great.

'Who'd like to go to the circus?'

'What sort of circus?' Didn't worry me, any sort of circus would be sensational, after all I'd worked as a young vet with the Moscow Circus when it played in Sydney.

The ballet was the Bolshoi, and performed in their very own Moscow venue. The performance was absolutely awesome. Seated in the third row, you know what Les Hiddings says, 'Doesn't get any better than this', he was right, and it was *Swan Lake*, to boot! The circus night proved to be just as unbelievable. Juggling, conjuring, acrobatics, animals, just amazing stuff, the ring was never empty and regardless of language barriers the clowns were sensational. Seats in the second row, how good is this? In life you need to take a gamble; only four of us went, the other six still regret it to this day!

Sundays are a day of rest, or so it was for most people in the city; for we animal nuts it was a chance to visit the Moscow pet market. We knew its location to be a huge open-air car park. It takes a lot of organising to get to an event like this simply because it's off the normal agenda and guides seem a little reluctant to allow tourists to depart from the accepted protocols. Once again good old US currency talks all languages and there we were, courtesy of a taxi, dumped at the market. Everyday people, with their animals. This is what I'd come to see and it was fantastic. It doesn't matter where you live, anywhere on this planet, if you love animals you'll have no trouble finding other people with the same love and interests. There were birds by the hundreds, budgerigars of all the colours and varieties that we were used to back home. Surely this little bird must be our most popular export. They hung from rickety stands in tiny little cages, many of which were handmade from wire, scraps of wood and metal, soldered or welded or twisted together in artistic and at times simplistic patterns. There were thrush, goldfinches and some species I'd never encountered before, but all were small, nothing resembling our larger parrots or cockatoos. The odd fancy pigeon and two or three different doves were about as big as the cage birds got. Plenty of poultry were for sale: bantams, ducks, a few geese and guinea fowl. Individual people seated on boxes or stools were selling one or two birds, perhaps just one chicken, or one small nesting box. No pet shops as we know them. So many people, each one intent on making an extra rouble or two for their week, pleading with the passers-by to make a purchase. Further along, wondrous old ladies with weather-worn faces, framed by thick woollen shawls tied around their heads and with heavy tattered overcoats hanging awkwardly on their shoulders, sat behind low wooden tables. Spread out in front of them were a dozen or more tiny little bags. Some were paper, some hessian, and each one brimmed full with a special seed. These were not the commercial seeds of aviculture, not just millets and canary, wheat and oats. These were seeds they had collected by hand. Each special wild seed was carefully measured and sold by the teaspoonful. I had no idea what these seeds were and regrettably no one could tell me. Each portion, carefully wrapped in folded newspaper, was stuffed inside a colourless shopping bag. These were the special treats for their own feathered friends. Russians love their birds. In row after row sat these enchanting, yet ancient, faces, all haggling and cajoling their customer to purchase perhaps just one more spoonful of this seed or that.

It doesn't take much imagination to picture these ladies spending their week collecting these seeds from the weeds and plants that grow along the lanes and pastures of their farmland. Taking them home, carefully drying and separating each individual grain to present their merchandise in the most favourable light. It seems that in the midst of so much emphasis on collective farming and the good of all, there is still room for independent income, no matter how small.

Ever seen a nutria? It is a huge rodent-like animal – we'd already encountered one at the circus conjuring act some two nights previously. They're almost as big as a cat, and look exactly like a dark brown rat. You could buy these too, but heaven only knows what you would do with them. There were dogs, even a couple of pure breeds: poodles and Pomeranians, but not very many cats. There were plenty of purchasers, business was brisk, lots of roubles changing hands. Two hours there were not enough, pictures these days stir the memory, but the train to Leningrad waits for no one and it was time to leave.

Leningrad, or St Petersburg as it is now known again, is every bit the romantic city that tourist brochures would have us believe. Magnificent architecture, art galleries, sculptures and the like, make a visit there very worthwhile. It was here that we all split up. Most would travel back home via Europe and Asia. We would go on to England and a motor holiday around Europe. Climbing aboard our final Soviet jet for the flight to London, we left with mixed emotions. The Soviet Union was just so big and so diverse, its population likewise, both in ethnic customs and in terms of prosperity. There had been so much to see in so little time. To go back is a must, for certainly much will have changed in the years since then. Strange, though, how some things have a habit of reappearing.

The huge jet roared down the airstrip and up through the clouds. This was an Aeroflot international flight. We had a couple of hosties. There would even be some in-flight service. Such anticipation. We had never encountered Soviet airline food. It arrived on a tray, in a box. A cardboard box!

It was only a fortnight ago, while travelling on Australia's own domestic airline, that I experienced a certain déjà vu.

'You know,' I said to the purser on the flight, 'we have been very slow to catch up to the Russians.'

'What do you mean?' he asked.

'Well,' I explained, 'I flew on Aeroflot well over twenty years ago, they had cardboard boxes back then.'

'Did they?' he exclaimed.

'Yes, they did, but you guys have gone one better . . . the food these days tastes better than the boxes.'

Or does it?

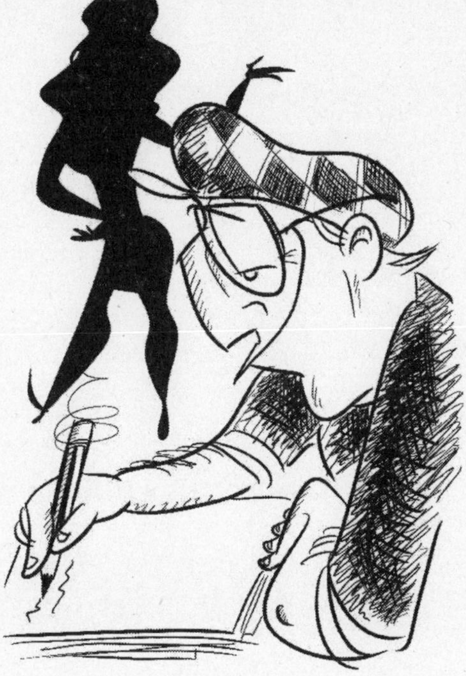

Janine's Stories

For the last eighteen years of my life it's been my great pleasure, and admittedly sometimes a little painful, to have been partnered by a woman whose love of animals one could only measure in armfuls. My darling wife was born 22-5-50 so that makes her about six years behind me as far as age is concerned but about twenty-five ahead in commonsense.

After the separation and divorce from my first wife, she appeared like some angel out of the blue, but an angel who came with something of an entourage of horses, dogs and cats. I've written elsewhere of how we came to meet and of how two failed partnerships led to the establishment of one that is still going strong and getting stronger seventeen years down the track.

Initially there was the euthanasia of her poor goat, badly savaged by an uncontrollable boxer, a neighbour's dog from just down the road. Billy was the goat's name. He was nothing special, just a neutered feral from the Northern Territory, but this somewhat different pet had been with her for quite a while. Trucked down from up north to be run through a saleyard in eastern Victoria, he'd been a poor, miserable specimen of a thing, too skinny for anyone to even raise a bid when she rescued him. With her kindness and good tucker, he'd become a bit of a character, following her around the place very much like a dog. Billy was used to being tethered, so while she rented here and there on her travels around eastern Australia, the goat followed, seemingly quite at home while sitting up on the back seat of the Kingswood.

At the time she lived in a rental property only three doors down the road from my veterinary practice in Annangrove. We'd never actually met. She hid inside the house and watched through a curtain while I did what had to be done and took the poor animal back home to bury it in the back garden. Next, there were the two budgies that I didn't mind looking after while she whizzed off with the love of her life, to a not-so-good life on a mine site in Queensland. Almost six months later we were to meet again, this time it was another euthanasia, a German Shepherd cross pup that had turned nasty and couldn't be confined inside her yard.

'What are you doing back here?' I asked. 'What happened to the love of your life?'

'You know how things don't always work out the way you plan,' she replied with a somewhat downward inclination of her head. Yeah, I knew.

'I've been married nearly fifteen years and it's all about to fold.'

'We should have a cup of coffee and talk about it sometime,' she said.

'Give us your phone number.' Fancy chatting up a bird after you've been with another woman for twenty years; it took two weeks to make the phone call.

We met once or twice over the next month for a meal and a real heart-to-heart. It was pretty obvious right from the word go: this woman was even more passionate about animals than I was. So followed the divorce, the settlement and, worse still, the custody arrangements for the children. Divorce is a bastard, there's no other word to describe it. It's worse than death and almost as bad as moving. Eventually things settle down and you get on with life. Don't look back, always look forward, but profit from those experiences of the past. We have tried to do that in our lives together, there have been plenty of downs, particularly the heartbreaking losses at Mole Creek (I talked about our time there in *Remedies & Memories*), but then again rather than break us, they probably made our marriage stronger.

These stories are Janine's stories and if they appear a little second-hand, then that is exactly what they are. Stories told to me over the years and tales that I will retell to you now on her behalf. She will read them, she will edit them and knowing my wife as I do, probably make some dramatic changes. They are hers, nevertheless, and provide some insight, I believe, into the success that we have had not only in life, but in exhibiting and breeding all manner of livestock. Utilising our home, our farm, our animals and ourselves as a medium to educate and entertain through that wonderful format called television has been both a trial and a pleasure at once. Yes, my friends, without my wife, there would be no Dr Harry.

28

The Beginning

Janine's early childhood was not quite what you would expect of someone who now looks after such a lot of animals. Up to the age of six she lived with her parents in a modest flat in North Sydney. Even in those days the area around her was densely populated with houses on every spare block of land, parks were at a premium. Still, from the age of four she managed to adopt a stray kitten whose poor mum had abandoned part of a litter on the back doorstep of the unit. Her early childhood books still gather dust in an old cabin trunk tucked under a desk in my office, and our daughter Heidi as a child herself enjoyed such wondrous publications as *Pitter Pat the Tabby Cat* and *Little Trotty the Pony*. As I've said so often, you start off in life the way you mean to finish. From the age of six onwards, life became a good deal more adventurous for Janine as the family moved to a large block in Turramurra.

In the late 1950s the upper north shore of Sydney was nowhere near as closely settled as it is today. The houses were large and the blocks even larger, every weekend was spent on the building site as the family home rose from humble foundations to the solid brick edifice that still appears today. With room to move and wildlife in abundance, Janine was to live and grow in an area where at last her animals had the freedom and the environment so necessary for their wellbeing.

Childhood pets were many and varied. Silkworms were just the beginning, as they were for so many of us back in those days; they cost virtually nothing to buy and if there was a mulberry tree nearby to provide all that the little caterpillars needed for their survival, then keeping them was a cinch. The old shoe box with a few holes punched in the lid, a regular supply of leaves and that anxious wait for the first cocoon to be spun with that beautiful silk. Then there's the trick of finding where the thread starts on the cocoon, as it bobs up and down in a bowl of water, while you try to spin the golden yarn onto a rectangular piece of cardboard with a dolly clothes peg on each side, making it easy to spin the device between thumb and finger of each hand. None of your fancy looms, kids couldn't afford that stuff and, besides, once you'd spun two or three cocoons onto the cardboard, you could cut it in half, knot it in the middle and it made a fabulous bookmark, just the ideal present for Grandma at Christmas. Of course we had to spare at least half a dozen cocoons and allow them to hatch into those awkwardly cumbersome moths that would stagger around all over the dead leaves laying eggs wherever they pleased. The biggest problem of the whole exercise was to remember to put some leaves in again once the eggs hatched, so most children's experience with these now-forgotten insects was limited to one breeding season and one only. Not Janine's – hers went on for years!

Then there was the frog. Most of us as kids on our way home from school or on a weekend outing could always find a pool or two, or a shallow creek with a plentiful supply of tadpoles. To bring them home, nurture them and watch the amphibian develop legs and finally lose that tail was a lesson in development that was learned so naturally. Janine took it one step further, she kept a frog. A big green tree frog in a magnificently decorated tank, it perched on her bedside table. How one could put up with the noise of a frog all night, I wouldn't know. As I'm something of a snorer, she's probably been accustomed to such noise for the last forty years.

Keeping amphibians in those days was something of a rarity, not like it is now. She had to collect the food and maintain the cleanliness of the tank all on her own. That meant setting up a lamp at night to attract moths and other flying insects which could be gathered alive with a net and fed to the frog, none of your over-the-counter live food like today.

Dixie was a mouse, a little white mouse that lived in her very own cage – set up in the outside toilet, as a matter of fact, its regular position was on top of the cistern. She was a real pet and would go everywhere Janine went, in her pocket or tucked inside her shirt. Regrettably, mice don't seem to last all that long and Dixie finally joined that great mouseatarium in the sky. There were tears for days. The coffin was a specially lined wooden tea canister complete with satin and velvet trimmings and the burial ground was under a lovely pink azalea that adorned the path to the front door.

There were even two budgies (one followed the other fairly quickly as budgies have a habit of doing) both by the name of Sweetie. Diminutive green and yellow specimens that as a breeder I know to have been Pieds. Like most of these amusing little birds they were always full of happiness, and showered the family with all the entertainment, birdseed and feathers that budgerigars are capable of dispensing. They both talked and whistled in tune. Janine was their teacher, she had and still has a beautiful singing voice. It was probably her mother who acted as a guiding light in these early years. Her dad, like mine, was heavily involved in the shipping industry, leaving home in the early hours of the morning and returning well after dark. They didn't know the meaning of a forty-hour week then.

There were three cats as well. First there was Inky, the seventeen-year-old who finally passed away peacefully in his sleep one night. He had been a kitten adopted from a litter that the next-door neighbour's tabby female had produced. Janine was to share much of her youth with this loving cat, and he proved to be such a great motivator for her future exploits into the cat world. It's funny how so many people who these days breed and exhibit all varieties of animals started off with just the average pet shop purchase. There were other cats as well. Smokey and Snoopy moved in to join the family not too long after Inky's death. One was a solid grey, which we correctly call blue, and the other a pretty, smoky tabby. How do I know all this in so much detail? There are pictures, many pictures and every picture tells a story, there are just so many of them.

Death is something that all children with animals quickly learn about. Quite honestly, it's something that I feel prepares them for one of life's tougher experiences. Nothing lives forever. Mice and silkworms spend such a short time with us, we begin to understand what Disney's *The Lion King*'s 'circle of life' is all about. One generation dies and another one is born to carry on. But when death comes abruptly and unexpectedly, that leads to trauma that even adults have difficulty in understanding. The back yard at Turramurra was large, blocks in those days were over fifty metres deep, probably twice what they are today, and in the shade of a large peach tree Janine had set up a guinea pig enclosure. Guinea pigs are delightful little creatures, animated, always chattering away and, of course, always eating. In fact, left to their own devices, eating and breeding would be their only interests in life.

Imagine the trauma of arriving home from school to find your pets slaughtered and lying in tattered remnants around the back yard. Janine can't tell me the names of those little rodents, but she can remember the name of the rotten dog from down the road that killed them, it was a big ugly cattle cross bitch called 'Jenny'.

A child of twelve who has painstakingly built the home for her precious animals with love and hard work must have been devastated.

'Can you remember it?' I asked her. 'How did it feel? And how do you feel now?'

'I cried for days, can you imagine picking up all the little bits and pieces of the animals that I loved so much and burying them in a communal grave? Mum and Dad went down and saw the people. I thought then and I still think now that the dog should have been put down.'

I can relate to this sort of thing, having seen dogs kill two of my own children's rabbits. There is no excuse, there will never be any excuse for this sort of behaviour. It behoves every one of us who owns an animal to make sure that this creature does not in any way cause problems for or damage to the environment or to the society in which we live. The dog control Acts that are being enforced today are in many ways not strong enough! No dog should ever be outside its front fence unless on a lead, or in a specially designated lead-free area and, heaven knows, we need more of those.

Did this make Janine hard? Did it make her vengeful? I believe the answer to all of this is no. She has become philosophical about people and the way they manage their stock. But that doesn't stop her from venting that sometimes acid spleen on the hapless or perhaps thoughtless individual who is basically doing the wrong thing with an animal.

29

Coco

Some horses are special, some horses unique – neither word could sum up Janine's Coke. He was something else. I didn't get to meet him until she'd actually moved in and at that stage he was in his late twenties, but let's go back to the beginning, as Janine tells the story.

Their yard in Turramurra backed onto the yard of a neighbour who had more than a passing interest in horses. His name was Frank Pickard. One of those people who just has an amazing ability to handle a horse. I've seen him in action as a much older man, but somehow you never really lose that ability, you're just a bit more careful in applying it. Frank worked for a major floating company called Livestock Transport. They carted horses hither and thither all over New South Wales and beyond. It didn't matter whether they were mares en route to a stallion or racehorses off to the track, Frank was their man. Occasionally it was the New South Wales Mounted Police that Frank was driving for, ferrying their tall bay geldings to agricultural shows and special events where the 'mounties', as they were affectionately known, would perform. This for Janine was manna from heaven, I think my wife loves horses more than any other animal.

Family holidays to Currarong on the south coast of New South Wales saw her learning to fish with her father, but more importantly, spending time at the local tip. It was here that the wild horses came to feed on the bread and scraps that were dumped by contractors and locals alike. By the end of a holiday not only had she managed to catch and lead one of these 'wild' ponies, but she damn well rode it as well. Children have no fear, this is perhaps their greatest attribute when dealing with horses. To Janine, it seemed a perfectly natural thing to do, she'd seen people ride, she couldn't afford a horse, but she could ride one of these, they cost nothing, just a loaf or two of bread to get one close enough to catch.

Frank was a sort of second father to Janine and at every opportunity she'd climb on board for a trip to wherever – as long as there were horses, she'd go. He taught her plenty, not the stuff you read in books, but the stuff that's passed down from generation to generation and from person to person. The way you move when you're around an animal, the approach, the retreat, your hands, your touch, even the way you use your eyes. It was on a trip to the Widden Valley, just out of Scone, that Janine first met Coco.

Scone today is still a major area for thoroughbred breeding in New South Wales. The lush pastures and fertile soils of the upper Hunter make it ideal and it's here that some of the best stallions in the land still stand. Frank had a load of mares on board bound for Alf Ellison's 'Barramul' stud. Alf stood 'Star Kingdom' and his outstanding son 'Todman'. These are legendary names even today and as a young vet it'd been my experience to vet the mighty Todman on more than one occasion.

Frank always introduced Janine as his daughter and in a sense, as I've said previously, she was certainly very close to this. You can imagine the stud with its white painted fences and long driveway leading down to the stables and the shedding. Coco and Coffee looked a little bit out of place amongst all these towering thoroughbreds: you see, Coffee was a buckskin and Coco was a skewbald, a Pinto in today's language. You'll remember the song about 'Old skewbald', who was a racehorse and never drank water, only drank wine (Peter Paul and Mary, I think). His colour was best described as white with patches of palomino: unusual, sure; pretty, yes! Coco had only one problem, he was ten years old and no one could ride him.

Thoroughbred studs use small pony stallions as so-called 'teasers' to detect when mares are in oestrus and ready to be served. Very often at the end of each season they mate these stallions with one or two crossbred mares to produce ponies for riding. Coke and Coffee were two of these, but it was only Coke that intrigued Janine.

'Could I have a go at him, Frank?' the young horsehandler asked.

'Geez, I dunno,' said the stable foreman, 'no one's been able to stay on his back, we tried breaking him to harness, but he demolished the jogger the first time we took him out. Not much future for this horse, I reckon.'

Frank spoke up. 'I'd like to take him back and have a go, if you don't mind.'

They didn't mind and so one horse made the return trip to Sydney and that was to be the start of a marvellous partnership.

Initially Frank worked with the horse at home, for they, too, had a big back yard and a couple of stables to house a pony or two. Janine would sit on the fence and watch for hours as he spent unresponsive days trying to gain the confidence of this gold and white pony.

'Couldn't I have a go, Frank?' she pleaded.

'He's got too much go for you, kiddo!' Frank casually threw back at her.

'But I could ride him, Frank, please let me try.'

Like water dripping on a stone, it eventually wears a hole, and so Janine wore Frank down. By this time he'd at least managed to get a saddle on the horse, but once he threw one leg in the stirrup, the horse would be up in the air in no time.

She didn't get on to begin with; in fact, she didn't get on for a day or two, didn't even attempt it, just spent time walking round and round the horse, patting him, stroking him and talking to him. Three days down the track, as nonchalantly as you please, her left foot slid into the stirrup and she pulled herself up into the saddle as if it were a regular occurrence. The horse never moved. He just stood there, quiet, relaxed and totally at ease. She adjusted her seat, leant forward to stroke his neck, he swung that big gold head around, saw her on board and in an instant accepted that he was hers, and so it was that horse and rider became one. But hang on a minute, it wasn't her horse.

Next weekend there's an ad in the paper for a horse, a pinto and it's him, the price one hundred dollars. Doesn't sound much today, does it? Janine was in tears, she was seventeen, she had no money, and was still studying at a secretarial college having left a school she'd never really liked, and had no prospects either. Her dad came to the rescue and lent her the purchase price. Coke became hers. That's five dollars a week out of a salary that at first was only $21.70; it takes quite a while and a special sort of perseverance to pay off the debt.

Coke moved next door into Janine's back yard, and her dad built a yard and eventually a stable as well. The frustrating thing about animals is that they often fail to do what we expect them to. Over two long hot weekends in February Janine's dad slaved from sunup to sundown to erect the shelter. Hardwood is a strong but heavy timber and sheets of galvanised iron become red-hot in the summer sun, but finally the job was completed and all the family were out to inspect Coke's home. It didn't take long for the weather to turn nasty; a typical Sydney thunderstorm roared in over the mountains. Threatening rumblings in the distance warned of heavy rains on the way.

'We got that finished just in time by the looks of things,' advised Janine's dad. Only Coke didn't think so. Down came the rain with a vengeance, and Coke, who had been quietly standing in his shed, now proceeded to walk out into the open yard and stand in the torrential rain. There's no pleasing some animals, is there?

Coke stood only 14.3 hands high and yet he could out-jump the 16-hand hacks at St Ives and Ryde pony clubs. When it came to one-day eventing he was the king. For a little horse he had a lot of go. Coke didn't walk and he didn't trot, he was a horse with a very unusual gait. What horsey people refer to as an ambler. He shuffled along and in so doing gave a magnificently smooth ride. Janine campaigned him at pony clubs, he taught countless children to ride, including my first two. There's a picture in our bedroom 'three up', Janine and the two of them bareback on the old fella riding round a paddock with just a halter on his head.

He went everywhere with her, to Queensland, to Melbourne where she was to buy an ex-Melbourne Cup starter called Precedent, a much bigger and in some ways more versatile horse, but with a temperament far inferior to Coke's. He led up a Melbourne Cup field for all but the last three furlongs, finished fifth last; still, that's something, isn't it? Coke was a great asset in the time Janine spent working in stables on the Mornington Peninsula. She could lead two fiery thoroughbreds off the old fella and he would never bat an eye. Frank came to collect her in Queensland. Precedent was such an idiot he went to sleep in the truck and fell over, Coke had been on so many different transports it was an everyday exercise for him. Precedent moved on.

Back in Coke's yard at Turramurra the peaches were in season. A huge tree hung over one corner of the fence. This horse was something of a connoisseur when it came to fruit, he would arch his neck right up, mouth each peach carefully and picking only the ripe ones, he would gormandise on their flesh, saliva drooling from his mouth, and then carefully spit the seed to the ground.

Love me, love my dog – and my horse and my cat and whatever else I may choose to bring. That's how Janine and I started life together and it hasn't changed since. I'm never surprised to see a new animal on the scene when I return from a week or so's filming. No good complaining, God made the animals before he made us.

Coke moved in not too long after Janine; I don't really think the horse ever liked me much, he was about twenty-seven at the time.

'I can't get near him, darl,' I used to complain.

'He just doesn't like men,' Janine explained.

'Every time I walk into the paddock he just turns his bum to me.'

'Give him time, he was like that with my dad at first.'

She was right, with time he came round, but somehow I was just someone who was there to offer food and shelter, and our relationship was strictly platonic. Hers was as she says 'made in heaven'.

At thirty years of age Coke passed away. We were in America at a veterinary conference; I didn't tell her. Imagine knowing the old fella had developed a shocking pleurisy and pneumonia just ten days into our trip. We drove down the long concrete pavement that stretched from the road to the home at Annangrove.

'Could you stop at the gate for a minute,' Janine asked, 'I'd just like to say hello to Coke.' I pulled up the car and she got out, calling to the old horse. It was dark and getting cold. 'He always comes when I call.'

'He can't hear you any more.' I had to tell my wife that the real love of her life, the animal she adored more than anything else was no longer here. But he was, and always will be, for he's buried where he used to stand at the very top of the hill surveying his domain; there's a fence around and a beautiful tree still grows over his grave. The loss of this horse meant more to my wife than the loss of anything before or since, for theirs was a very special partnership.

'I have to have something to ride, Cheryl [her friend from Dural pony club] and I are off to look at some horses this afternoon.' It made sense, my kids had their ponies and were off to pony club and down the trails whenever possible. Janine really had nothing to ride, our horses were all a bit small.

It's now about 6.30 in the afternoon and my evening clinic is in full swing. There are birds and slow greyhounds everywhere. The parking lot is chockers. Janine and Cheryl draw to a halt in the middle of the orchard, she races in the door excitedly, barges straight in on a consultation.

'You should see what we've bought!' Yeah, I could hardly wait. 'He's a bay quarter horse and, boy, is he good!'

She's back out the door in a flash and from the window I can see them unloading what, to my mind, was the ugliest horse in God's creation. It may have been a quarter horse, and it may've been good, but it had a head like a half-eaten pie with sauce and a body to match.

'Don't you like him?' I'll save my comments until after the clients leave, I thought.

Half an hour down the track, the melee has subsided.

'I'll get on him and show you what he can do,' she assured an obviously very dubious husband. 'I paid twelve hundred for him.'

'You got touched.' She went to get on board. 'Hang on, what about your helmet.'

'He'll be right, he didn't put a foot wrong.'

'Yeah, but that was there and this is here. You wait till I get a helmet.' I'm really tough about that, I meant what I said.

'Here you go,' I said, passing up the familiar white skullcap, but she never even got to put it on before the horse went straight up in the air. Bloody hell!! She hung on till all four feet were back on the ground.

'If he's any good, I'll eat him,' I said, passing the helmet once again to my now somewhat more careful wife. He was no good and must have been full of dope when she bought him. The rotten thing bolted three times with her and would rear whenever he felt like it. We sold him two months later, couldn't get him off the place quick enough. The new owners liked him, too, in a small yard he could turn on a sixpence, out in the open some of the screws came loose.

Amber was a beautiful mare, a copper chestnut, it was a long drive to Condobolin to pick her up. But she was class, real class. Over the years, Janine through Frank and his transport business had come to know many of the 'mounties', particularly the tent-pegging team, and she'd often tell of their favourite trick. A tent would be erected in the middle of a showground and then as part of their tent-pegging demonstration they would ride in from four different sides and collapse the tent. She'd emerge from underneath, boy, wouldn't occupational health and safety have a problem with that today, back then it was just good fun. It was through the mounties that Janine found Amber. She was with us almost up until the time we left for Tassie. Her loss was a tragedy. Probably the second-worst thing ever to hit Janine. Something had happened to a gate latch – had it been left open, had the pony undone the catch, who will ever know? But both horse and pony found themselves on the middle of the road late one night. A speeding car misses the pony and ploughs into the mare's hind leg, snapping it off just below the hock.

I felt sick . . . but you do what you have to do . . . and you do it quickly.

People often ask why you can't fix a horse with a broken leg; the answer is simply that by taking weight on only three legs the leg opposite eventually gives way as well. Such a mighty animal, so much power and speed and yet so fragile when it comes to injury. I shall never forget that night, she stood so still and so resigned, the remnants of her hind leg dangling in the grip of what few tendons remained. You pray to God to take you away so that it never really happened. You pray that you could be anywhere but here. You have friends and they come when you need them. They were there in an instant and it was done. Amber is buried alongside Coke. Naturally enough, it's a liquidambar that grows over her resting place.

There was no horse for Janine to bring to Tasmania, all the ponies were under fourteen hands and far too small. There was old Cindy, a docile pony mare that belonged to Frank (now since passed away) that we adopted as a sort of a keepsake and she'll be with us till she passes on too. This gentle chestnut lady foundered once or twice early in her life. Ponies have a habit of doing this. Food to them is an absolute necessity and too much good tucker impacts on their feet, producing a condition called laminitis (or founder). They become extremely lame and often suffer problems later in life as a result. Janine had broken her in as a two-year-old, and in an emergency, she will do as a mount. Her feet remain permanently affected, so she's a little stilted in her gait.

Trooper was an ex-racehorse, a big, rangy thoroughbred, but quiet as a lamb. Vern, who had brought our horses initially to Tassie, bought him for her. Trooper was a great horse and Janine had many a good time riding up into the high country near Mole Creek over the Christmas holidays with our dear friend and neighbour Dot's children and grandchildren. To ride through the pristine environment of the Tasmanian wilderness areas, to spend nights sleeping in slab huts where trappers and snarers had lived through a long winter is something a lot of people would give their eyeteeth for.

Horses have to be fed and that means bags of this and that as well as bales of hay. In lifting a large bag of oats from the boot of a car Janine badly ruptured two discs in the lower part of her back. She spent some six weeks in and out of bed on massive doses of painkillers with regular medical and chiropractic supervision. For half of this period she had no sensation in either leg and there were thoughts that she'd never walk again.

So Trooper moved on, and today, much as Janine would like to climb aboard again, her better judgment suggests she stays on the ground. What do I think about that? Well, I think one day she'll ride again. You get to a time in your life when priorities change, when your love of something you've held so dear for so long becomes seemingly more important than your own safety. She'll do it . . . don't ask me to, though . . . Yours truly looks pretty ordinary on a horse.

30

The Dogs and the Cats

Janine came with two dogs: a lovely old German Shepherd called Kushla and a diminutive blue cattle dog called Shandy. The Shepherd was a pound dog. Janine bought her at about five years of age, desexed, of course, and with a temperament that was extraordinary, nothing worried the old dog, not even the annoying interference of the cattle pup could rouse any sense of anger. She'd just follow along quietly behind wherever we went and when she'd had enough simply sit down somewhere in the shade of a tree and watch us. We'd always come back. I diagnosed her with heartworm disease not too long after she arrived, poor old girl, she had a dose and a half and never really recovered from the treatment. Still, I think without any therapy her life span would have been much less. Shocking hips and low spinal arthritis took her from us at the age of about ten. But she'd had a great life and whatever she missed in the first half Janine made up for in the second.

I've written about Shandy elsewhere and her demise at the hands of a brown snake. What a lovely little dog she was, always happy, always pleased to see you, the sort of dog that didn't just wag its tail, but wagged its whole body. She was a local product, bred down in the valley behind the Annangrove property. She spent most of our early courtship and marriage throwing up in the back seat of one car or another.

Janine did make one valiant effort to become involved in

pure breeds. At great expense we purchased a German Shepherd of almost entirely imported blood, her name was Karla. What a dead loss she turned out to be. Nice sort of a dog, but we put her in pup on her second season, had everything prepared for the imminent birth. A whelping box, heat lamp, bedding, etc, were all there. What did she do? Went for a quiet stroll around the back yard and under the clothesline, squatted as if to evacuate, dropped out a pup and simply walked away. We were left to rear the darned thing, she had not the slightest interest in anything maternal. That was the beginning and end of Janine's canine breeding activities. I'd better qualify that. For the time being.

Janine spent many years in southern Queensland in the area around Murwillumbah. It was cane country and she had regular employment at the local plumbing shop. Things get a bit lonely when you're living on a property and your only home is a caravan. Her partner at the time was fairly busy in his own endeavours, working long hours, often at weekends as well. She thought a cat would make a worthwhile companion and sought out a lady by the name of Faye Spher who owned a cattery at Fingal, not all that far away. She chose a cat entitled 'Fingali Blue Elysia', a blue-point Siamese female born 1974. She would prove to be a marvellous companion and went by many names, Lisa, Louie, Louie Bum-Fly and other such endearing terms as Janine would use from time to time, but the cat seemed to know them all. Janine became hooked on Siamese cats and decided somewhat prematurely that breeding them would be her particular thing. She became a member of the local cat club. In later years she would become secretary and then president of a Victorian cat club.

Faye had a seal-point Siamese stud cat called 'Arwen

Quicksilver' that had been imported from New Zealand, and offered the cat to Janine as a stud. She'd often admired him, and secretly believed that the cat didn't like Faye and vice versa as he'd gone for her on more than one occasion. Entire male cats can be a bit of a handful, they only need to smell the odour of another male on your clothing or your hands and they go off like a packet of crackers. This cat loved Janine and in no time a pen had been built and cats were being bred.

Moving from Queensland to the Mornington Peninsula was almost as big an undertaking for Janine as it was for us later to move to Tasmania from Sydney. She took with her two horses, and something like five cats. Circumstances down there were somewhat different and the stud cat had to find a new home in Melbourne. Most of the others were sold, except Lisa and a stunning neutered male called Kristen. Breeding activities ceased and both cats now became her fondest pets. Over time our attitudes change and for the second time in her life Janine found herself heading back to the security of the family home in Turramurra. It was from here that she would move to the mine site in Queensland – and that was no place for a cat.

Sally and Janine had been friends for years. Sally had the answer to Janine's woes.

'I've got a doctor friend, he lives just out of town.' This town being Albury. 'And he and his wife would be only too happy to take Kristen and Lisa,' so that's where they went. Quite a sacrifice really to unload two pets who'd been so close to you for so long, to someone who really was a total stranger, but then again, Janine had found the love of her life. Hadn't she? All I'd got was the two budgies!! . . . remember?

Poor Lisa the cat became totally disorientated, as animals do in strange circumstances. One morning she couldn't be found, the family searched high and low, but eventually it was time for the good doctor to leave for work, a drive of some forty minutes into town. Once parked in the hospital car park he headed for his rooms to begin afternoon consultations. It was a scorching summer's day, the midday temperature exceeded 40 degrees centigrade. Within thirty minutes a crowd had assembled around his vehicle in the car park. Strange noises were coming from under the bonnet and they certainly didn't sound remotely like a motor purring. It was a high-pitched continual scream, something or someone was in dire trouble . . . there was a knock on the doctor's door.

'Something's wrong with your car, John,' a courteous orderly informs him. 'Better come and have a look.'

By now the crowd had grown to twice its original size and the howls were becoming louder. There under the bonnet was poor little Lisa, jammed so rigidly beneath the exhaust manifold that most of the hair had been burnt from her back. A mechanic had to be summoned to disassemble a large part of the motor to release the cat. Cats have a habit of climbing up into warm areas and vehicle motors are just that. She'd travelled all the way into town hanging on to God knows what while her back was being burnt by the exhaust. Lisa survived the ordeal, and she healed. Janine's mine site relationship did not survive and she would soon pack up and leave. Daytime temperatures there were even hotter!

'Better come down here straight away,' said Sally on the phone. 'Lisa's gone missing again and they can't find her anywhere.' Janine was in Albury in a flash.

She spent four hours combing the property. Fifty acres is a lot of ground to cover. The cat had been gone four days. Was it a snake? It usually is. She searched the grounds where they'd last seen her. For hours she called and called, with tears in her eyes and a heavy heart weighed down with the guilt of having left such a very special animal. Life makes us all face decisions; we don't always make the right ones. Driving away was hard enough, leaving behind forever this time her very special cat was just too much. She went back and called again around the house in particular and behind the garage. No result. Darkness set in. Back at Sally's home in town there was no consoling her. 'It's all my fault, I've lost her and she'll never be back, there'll never be another Lisa.'

It's 5.30 the next afternoon, Janine's preparing for the drive back home to Turramurra.

'They've found her . . . they've found her!' screams Sally through the open window. In an instant Janine is out the drive and heading for the farm, yelling instructions as she goes.

'Tell 'em to lock her up, don't let her out.'

'Take her back, Janine, take her back with you – she's your cat, she could never be anyone else's. Kristen can stay, he's happy here, but Lisa should go with you.'

Who would know where she'd hidden those four days and how far away she had gone, but the voice so familiar and so tearful had called her back, and once again Janine and Lisa were together.

And so I came to meet Lisa, probably the most important cat ever to grace our doorstep. She had some funny habits. I believe right from the word go, even though it was my home, and her mother had moved in with me, Lisa thought that still gave her the right to take over the entire joint. She even slept on the end of the bed, something none of our cats do any more. There was no intimidating this animal, in fact, it was just the reverse. There we'd be lying in bed on a Sunday morning or whenever, and I would simply lean over to give my darling a little cuddle.

This damned cat would physically intrude between the two of us, placing both front feet deliberately on either side of my neck and staring directly into my eyes as if to say, 'What do you think you're doing to my mother?' In the end we had to lock her out of the bedroom and then put in the earplugs!

We got into cat breeding via a trip to Surfers Paradise. It was bucketing down rain again, it always did when we went there. Our unit was close to the beach, a ground-floor job with a really good occupancy rate. We'd go up in October and the locals would say, 'You should be here in November, the weather's always better.' So next year we'd do just that and get drowned again. 'Oh! You should have been here in October, it was sensational . . .' We couldn't win, so we sold it. On one of these miserable holidays, having spent all we could in the local boutiques, I asked, 'Why don't you give Faye a ring, she still breeds cats, doesn't she? She might know of some we can look at.' She did.

We travelled south a bit to look at some Burmese. I liked them right from the word go. Now, the lady had a blue/cream female with a litter of kittens, they were just gorgeous. 'Gee, I'd like to get a kitten out of the same litter next time you breed them.' The lady nodded in acknowledgment. So here we are again twelve months down the track and it's raining yet again. The decision's made, we'll ring this woman and see if she's home.

'Hello, do you remember me?' She did. 'Could we come down and have another look, do you have any kittens for sale?'

'Yes,' she said, 'they're all for sale.' Good, I thought, we'll be able to pick one.

Our cat breeder was quick to open the door when we knocked. 'Please come in, they're all for sale.'

'Yes, but we only want to buy one,' I assured her.

'Yes,' she said, 'but they are all for sale.'

'What do you mean, they're all for sale?'

'My husband and I are splitting up and I want to get rid of all the cats.' At this stage I suspected she needed to get rid of them in one hell of a hurry and probably stash the loot in her pocket (voice of experience).

'What do you reckon this lot's worth,' I asked Janine.

'Well,' she said, 'there's a stud cat, three Burmese queens, one with a litter of six and a Siamese queen as well.' She came up with a figure. I halved it.

'I'll give you xxx dollars cash money now and take the lot, you've got two minutes to make up your mind.' It took her thirty seconds.

'Don't move,' I told Janine, 'stay right here, I'll whiz over to the bank and get the cash.' When I returned all the cats were in baskets. The loot changed hands. The transfers were signed and we were out of there. 'For Pete's sake, don't tell her where we're staying, or where we live, for that matter.' They may have had second thoughts!

We drove home with most of them in the back of the car, but flew the stud cat home, he stank . . . And so it was that Sam, Bonnie, Mia, Tilly, her six kittens and the Siamese pushed the budgies out of two aviaries and our cat breeding program began. In time Quicksilver, or Flash, as we knew him, came home as well. It seemed that at last Janine's life was complete, she had her horses, she had her cats, she had her dogs and not too far down the track she had her child. Like so many pieces of a living jigsaw puzzle, we'd brought animals back to our fold and you know what? It felt good!

Lisa and Flash lie buried under the shade of a massive

willow on the creek banks of 'The Den' at Mole Creek. Bonnie was desexed and went to a pet home, as did the Siamese. Mia lived on in her familiar environment at Annangrove, passing away peacefully at sixteen years of age, so the new owners tell us. Sam was with us right through all our moves, he left us in our early days at Relbia. And Tilly, what of 'Chantilly Lace'; well, without her, I'd doubt we'd have half the good cats we've got today. She was our foundation, and between her and Sam we've managed to build a cattery and a reputation that we're proud of . . . Thanks, geez . . . I'm glad they were *all for sale*!

As I write there are three house cats. There's Tinkerbell, the snooty Siamese ('Don't pat the cat,' we have to warn visitors) and Gretel, whom you've seen from time to time on TV, direct from the local pet shop, she's a semi-longhair with beautiful ginger markings on a stunning white coat, she'd pass for a Turkish Van cat and looks better than most that I've seen in recent times. Lastly, Shandy, named after guess who? An adventurous Maine coon, she's a silver tortie tabby with the longest tail and the fluffiest ears you've ever seen. They share the house with Isabelle and Tabitha, the two Italian greyhounds. In an outside run live Otis, my beautiful red Burmese; Lucky, a gorgeous Abyssinian (bred by Faye, just before her death and therefore terribly important); and Snoopy, our foreign white – all of whom spray like a firehose, hence their banishment from the house as such. We love them all.

31

Of Men and Mice

So, Janine and I hadn't been together all that long when the animal population of Annangrove began to undergo something of an explosion. First of all it was horses, Welsh and Australian ponies, then it was dogs, closely followed by the goldfish, but things didn't stop there. Young Russell, my son, had expressed a keen interest in getting something a little more interactive than a goldfish, and mice were chosen to fill the bill.

It's not just the mice you need, it's the wherewithal to go with it. This means a tank, absorbent material for the base, ladders, wheels and appropriate housing, then there's the food bill. It's never enough for our mice to live on a simple diet of seed and pellets, no . . . they need every other goody that a pet shop or supermarket can provide. From memory we started with two, but very quickly two become ten; as luck would have it, both of the females were pregnant.

'It's all part of his education,' I was assured by my darling wife. 'It's good for children to see animals being born and growing up.'

For a time the mice appeared to live quite happily in their little tank oblivious to whatever may have been going on around them, but suddenly the count changed. There used to be ten, now there's only seven – where are the other three? It was hard to tell exactly where they were, except to say they were somewhere in the room. Evidence would appear from time to time by way of droppings, shredded paper and some gnawing on the lid of the tank indicating their attempts to join their relatives in seeming luxury below. You'd open a draw and there would be a mouse nest, inside a cupboard there'd be another, the bludgers were everywhere, but you never got to see them. Hear them, yes; see them, no. We couldn't set ordinary mousetraps, fancy catching them and killing them, no one in the house would permit that. So they continued to live free-range, as it were, in the bedroom.

'Can you smell something?' Janine can always smell something, her nose is so much more sensitive than mine.

'Yeah, smells like something burning.' But we didn't have an open fire back then. Following the scent like a bloodhound, Janine rapidly homed in on Russell's room.

'It's in here for sure!' I had to agree. And what's more it seemed to be coming from near the bed. She flung back the covers. The smell was even more intense.

'That's smoke . . . there's smoke coming from the mattress!' I exclaimed, tearing the bottom sheet off the bed. Sure enough, there it was, a smouldering area some ten centimetres or so across. Janine went to have a close look. 'Don't touch it . . . That's the electric blanket!'

Having disconnected the blanket from the power socket behind the bedhead we heaved the thing holus-bolus from the bed. The rotten little rodents had found the warmest place in the whole room to make their bed and in so doing had chewed a great heap of insulation right off the electric cables within the blanket. How lucky were we? The whole joint could have gone up in smoke.

That was it for Janine – there'd be no more mice. They don't live long anyhow. The vast majority develop massive tumours which eventually become almost as big as the mouse, and you lose them. I've been a bit off mice ever since I had a hundred crawling all over me in a picture shoot to celebrate the one-hundredth episode of 'Talk to the Animals'. It took six washes to get the smell out of the clothes. Mice don't seem to have a proper bladder so they just drip urine all the time.

'We'll change them for some rats,' championed Janine, 'they don't smell – well, not quite as much and they've got a lot more brains.' She's certainly right about that part. We caught the lot in special harmless traps and traded them in forthwith.

It was only recently that one of my soundos had a similar problem. His darling wife had bought their daughter a mouse as a present and just like ours the little waif had been set up in a tank with all the accoutrements. There's only one problem: what one child in a family has, the other one wants as well, and so it was that he directed his darling to journey back to the same pet shop and buy another mouse that would not only keep the first one company, but could be the exclusive property of their son.

Children are always over anxious. 'He was so keen to get the darned thing home that ten minutes into the journey he opens the lid of the box and the darned mouse jumps out, and now it's in the car somewhere and we can't find it. What am I gonna do, Harry?' I explained in some detail that these traps can be bought which look like square lobster pots with an inverted cone in the top through which the mouse enters, but once in finds escape impossible. You simply bait the trap with a bit of birdseed or perhaps a piece of bacon rind.

Since we were on a filming trip at the time he's conveyed all these instructions by phone to his beloved back home. She is by now feeling somewhat ill-at-ease when driving her car. In short, the stench is becoming unbelievable – twice she sets the trap and twice the mouse escapes with the bacon rind.

'She needs to squeeze the cone together a bit more,' I advise.

She does that and the mouse stays away. She pleads to be able to drive his car. He refuses, with a grin that would put a Cheshire cat to shame.

Between them they decide there's only one thing for it, pet mouse or not it's got to be caught dead or alive before the car becomes a total write-off, for now the upholstery is being gobbled as well. The trap is set. The trap is sprung, triumphantly his wife strides to the car having heard the commotion through the open window, flings open the back door to find the mouse gasping its last in the trap. Feeling a pang of compassion she releases the spring to remove the poor animal and dispatch it humanely. The mouse gives one last dramatic convulsion and flips from her hand back into the car, where it disappears under the back seat to die in peace. The smell, my friends, is now ten times worse than it ever was and so far no one has managed to find the corpse . . . The moral of this story is . . . a live mouse always smells better than a dead one!

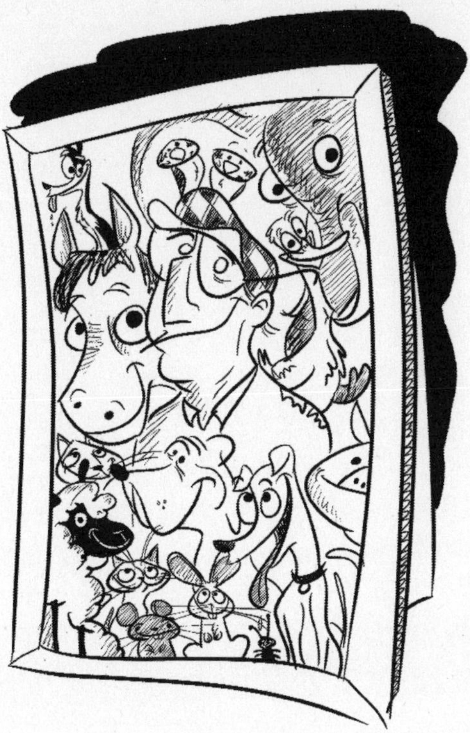

Life with Animals

32

More About Sheep

I've recounted elsewhere so many stories about our exploits with those woolly four-legged fruitcakes that you'd reckon there couldn't be too much more left to tell. Well, there is!

I can well remember Banjo Paterson in one of his poems talking about that well-known character Saltbush Bill the drover and his mob of 'lousy sheep'. To a city slicker the word lousy simply means pretty poor quality or skinny-looking when applied to animals, but out on The Den at Mole Creek we were to find out that lousy really did mean just what it said, not what I thought. A neighbour brought in a mob of sheep right next door and as animals will, our sheep got to know their sheep through the fence. Sheep are, after all, quite sociable animals. We should have woken up to things right from the word go.

'They're lousy sheep,' our mentor Dot advised of the mob that was now settling down alongside our boundary.

'Yeah, they don't look too good,' I replied.

'No,' she said, 'they've got lice. See that wool and just you watch them rubbin' up against all the fences.'

She was right – the more you looked at the poor damn animals the more they seemed to rub and scratch. That's what sheep infested with lice do. Rub on anything to relieve the irritation. The wool is next to useless.

Panic ensued. For over a week they'd been getting on

famously with our mob of 'clean' sheep. Horror. Now some of ours were rubbing too. As any parent with school-age children will know, lice are super-contagious!

We had bought at one stage a device called a jetting race. I will attempt to describe this elaborate apparatus. The actual race itself is about as long as two sheep, with solid walls on each side up to about chest height. Inside are two rows of spray jets on each side, which become activated by a bar that each sheep compresses as it walks through the system. A pump and vat supply the insecticide and the chemical is driven at high pressure right through that woolly topcoat to the skin beneath. The success or otherwise of this strategy depended on the lice going for a stroll for at least part of the day so that they might come in contact with at least some of the poison, deposited in two fairly narrow bands.

'Waste of time,' advised Dot, 'just don't get enough of the stuff in there to do any good. All right for flies but no good for lice.'

We're back at square one.

'OK then, what do you suggest we use?' I asked in a somewhat derisive fashion.

'The dip, of course.'

'But we don't have a dip.'

'Oh, yes you do.' Dot knew so much more about the place than anyone else in the district and I suppose she should because for most of her married life she had lived right next door. 'It's under all those brambles, down near the creek. Where those old yards are falling down. She'll need a bit of cleaning up but it's still a goer.'

Thank heavens for school holidays, all Dot's grandkids thought it would be top fun to get the old dip up and running again. They worked like slaves, shovelling and bucketing the silt from the bottom of the concrete trough. Fences were rebuilt, temporary yards installed with portable sheep panels, and the lot was ready to go in three days. The dip solution was mixed with water pumped from the creek and things were looking good. A dip is very different to a jetting race. This is a permanent in-ground structure, some four metres long and nearly a metre in width, and about a metre and a half deep. It's buried in the ground, very much like a miniature swimming pool, but without all the fancy bits and pieces. The sheep don't just walk through the thing. They have to jump in and swim to the other end where there is a ramp to help them crawl out. Point number one. Most sheep don't like swimming. To overcome this problem one simply needs physical force. Easier said than done.

The first mob of around 300 are penned up and ready to go. Dogs are barking, kids are yelling and pushing, but one look at that lap pool and no sheep is going to take the plunge. Someone's got to do it. So the fittest and strongest are in there with the mob, dragging the first two or three protesting woollies towards the deep end. With a splash they're in, and sheep being as they are, followers rather then leaders, the rest soon begin to follow. Two or three helpers are on hand to make sure every poor ewe and wether on our entire property gets a complete dunking. Pushing sheep underwater with a long pole is just the best school holiday fun.

Over two days everything in sight got a good, thorough dipping. The operators, too, were inclined to get a spot of treatment. It was all in a day's work. Only one job remained: to dip the rams!

Janine and I had taken quite a liking to the Suffolk breed of sheep, and early on decided that we would become a 'daughter stud' to the best in Tasmania. This left us with a mob of nearly 100 head of which thirty-odd were rams. Some were our stud breeding fellas and the others were so called 'flock rams' that we mated with our border/Merino cross and Polwarth ewes to produce our spring lambs each year. Suffolk are a British breed of sheep. Suffolk are big, strong sheep. Ours were bigger and stronger than most, as they were from American imported blood. Each ram weighed well over sixty kilos. They were massive, mean and downright cranky. To get them into the dip was something else. They would try to hurdle the whole thing. They would try to creep along one edge. They would charge at any operator or any dog that looked like being a threat. Half the staff ended up in the dip with the rams! But finally and triumphantly they all got done. Janine reckons she copped enough insecticide to vermin-proof her for life!

When we sold the Mole Creek property the Suffolks went too, to another small stud somewhere west of Mole Creek. Dot took the very best of our young border/Merino crosses and even now, some ten or more years down the track, she still has three. They twin every year. Often when we visit out Mole Creek way and enjoy a barbecue beside the little creek that bears the same name, we talk about the good times on The Den, and the time we dipped the rams. It's all filled in now. Not environmentally sound, you know, but back then we'd never have managed without it.

33

Northern Memories

Since the early days of 'Harry's Practice' we have spent a lot more time out on the road. As the show screens all over this wonderful country of ours we thought it only right that we should make sure we attempt to traverse as much of Australia as possible, answering questions and solving problems as we go. I enjoy the contact with people, the challenge that every new case brings, particularly the behaviour-orientated problems. Very often there's the bonus of a chance to catch up with old friends. Such was the case on a recent visit to northern New South Wales.

In what I like to refer to as my previous life, my wife and I had spent many wonderful holidays fishing in and around the Clarence River. It was quite ridiculous when you come to think of it. We'd be up well before sunrise every morning, breakfast in a hurry, grab the sandwiches we'd made the night before and race down to the boat ramp where our trusty aluminium punt would be dragged from the roof of the car, the outboard attached and we'd race across the ebbing tide to our favourite spot on the middle wall. Often it was underwater when we got there, but the best fish were to be had as the tide fell, and there was great competition amongst the fishing fraternity for the best spots. First in, more chance of getting a feed. We always got that. Yamba was renowned for blackfish!

They are a cunning fish. You need all the right equipment. Light line, carefully balanced float and sinkers, well-greased line to sit on the water and the knack of knowing just when to strike at a rapidly disappearing float. All this is learnt. The real key to success was the bait. These fish are weed eaters. If you have the right weed you'll have a great day. If you don't, then better pack it in before you start. On the days before the trip I'd scour the foreshores of the Parramatta River for the many and varied types of green weed. Some years they liked the coarse dark stuff, other times it would be the really fine yellow forms. Like a good boy scout you needed to be prepared. Most days we could hook around fifty. On the best days, try eighty! All were big fish, no little stuff here. Even after the birth of our first daughter we were still at it.

Only six months old, but safe in her own life jacket, Tiffany would lie in her carrycot in the bottom of the boat, which was kellicked on the smooth water side of the wall, while the two of us fished the rough. This day the place was packed. Blokes and rods everywhere. The two of us were hauling them in. Big bronze sea luderick, very different to the river fish. No one else was doing much good. Then this bloke a few yards on the seaward side of me strikes up a conversation.

'Don't seem to be able to get a down.'

'What weed have you got?' I asked, intent on netting another struggling beauty from the very edge of the oyster-covered rocks. 'Gotcha!'

'Oh, this is just some local weed from down near the old boatshed,' he replied.

'Well, this is Putney weed we've got,' I said. 'We bring it up from Sydney every year.'

Just then my wife interrupted. 'Could you mind my rod for a minute?' Since I was in the process of unhooking my fish and popping it into the swimmer to keep it alive till the day's end, I just leant over and grabbed the tip. She went back to the boat, picked up our bub, carrycot and all. Placing the wicker cradle carefully between two of those razor-sharp rocks, she picked up the bub and began to feed her. 'Pass us back the rod, will you?'

I did. That very minute she hooked a fish. No problem, with the baby perched carefully on her lap, she proceeded to play the piscean performer for all it was worth. It took a good three minutes before another beautiful fish lay quietly in the water at her feet. I netted the fish.

'Bloody hell!' says the bloke next door to me. 'Did you see that woman? She's feedin' a kid and fishin' all at the one time and I'm not even getting a touch.' He would have gone home empty, too, if we hadn't chipped in half a dozen of ours to fill out his bag.

When our second child arrived things had to change. We said goodbye to Yamba and elected instead to travel each year to Wooli, just a bit farther south, but for a different reason. Every August the city of Grafton hosts a huge racing carnival. Horses and greyhounds from all over the place congregate for what is both fabulous racing and a great social event. We would take enough equipment from the Annangrove surgery with us, and the boat, and rent a house right on the beach so the kids could play while I tried to sort out what had gone wrong with this dog and that in last night's racing. We could X-ray, operate, the lot! Clients came from as far as Melbourne, but many were my regulars from Sydney anyhow. Four hours every morning looking at dogs and the rest of the day was ours. Fishing, walking and often a visit to the gallops, or the dogs at night. The holiday always paid for itself.

Here it is a Saturday in May 2002, and I find myself trying

to sort out a misbehaving little Australian terrier. It's only ten minutes' drive down the road to Iluka, a sleepy township on the northern side of the mighty Clarence River. Yamba is on the other side. You wonder how much things have changed. Is the boat ramp in front of the old wooden pub still there? It's where we'd come for a beer and I'd clean the day's catch. The mossies were so bad they'd bite you through the seat of your trousers. In the hurly-burly world of television can I spare an hour to relive a memory? I can and I do, and I know having done it I must do it more often. Yes, the pub is there. It's raining in buckets so that's a good excuse to have a feed of fish and chips. What else would you eat in a place like this?

Friends from Sydney moved here. They once owned some flats near the water. Were they still here too? It's seventeen years ago. They are. We enjoy a cuppa and more memories come flooding back.

Their son was a builder and a damn good one at that. He was also a dead keen budgie breeder. Being around ten years younger than me, and a lot more capable when it came to construction, he was in charge of adding on a whole new section to my aviaries at Annangrove. Thinking back it was probably twenty-five years ago. Some friends had arrived and I'd left him to it for an hour to have a quick coffee with them. Back on the job, he had me up on the roof walking along some struts he'd nailed in place whilst I was away. 'Careful, Harry. Only every second one will take your weight.' Trouble was, I didn't know where to start counting. In an instant my right foot steps onto an unsupported beam, and it and I crash two metres to the concrete floor below.

'I've broken me bloody arm,' I gasp in some early state of shock.

'How do you know it's broken?' he asks in a rather awkward fashion.

'Well, I can't usually get me left arm up behind me back to scratch me bloody ear, can I?' Now he believes me. 'Roll me over,' he looks paler than I feel. 'Pull my arm out from behind my back.'

'Are you sure?'

'Of course I'm bloody sure!' Slowly he eases the arm out from underneath me and lays it by my side. 'Now grab a bit of two-be-one and pull my arm out straight.'

'You're kidding!'

'No, I'm not kidding . . . just bloody hurry up.' The pain was beginning to start, and if he didn't get a wriggle on I'd be in agony. 'Right . . . put your foot against my chest and pull hard on my wrist.' Working now like a complete automaton, he did. I grabbed at the middle of the left forearm and squeezed like hell. The bones grated and seemed to straighten. 'OK, strap the timber to the arm while you've got it stretched and we'll get to hospital.'

Emergency ward sisters are all the same. 'What's your problem?' she asked in an almost totally removed fashion.

'I've broken my arm,' I recited quite calmly and politely.

'That's for the doctor to decide,' she said abruptly. 'Take a seat.'

After the usual two-hour wait, the room filled with the noise of crying babies, sobbing mothers, alternating with the sound of coughing and vomiting, it's finally my turn. In the examination room a pleasant young female doctor asks me the nature of the problem.

'I've got a mid-shaft fracture of the left humerus,' I spout with all the confidence of over ten years as a vet.

'Take off that splint and that jumper.' That was no easy task, particularly when left to do it on your own. Fainting was a near thing! She grabbed the upper arm with both hands and gave it a twist.

'Aaaa . . . Bloody hell!!' Yes, it hurts.

'I don't think it's broken.'

'You must be bloody joking . . . what about the crepitus [bone crunching on bone]?'

'Oh, you get that with muscle injuries too.'

'How long have you been out?'

'What was that?' Thank heavens I'd mumbled.

'Nothing . . . just let's get an X-ray.'

'If you really want one.'

'Yes, I really do want one!'

'Sure enough,' says the radiologist, 'broken smack through the middle just like you said.' Thank heavens someone got it right. On went the heavy plaster.

'It's lovely and straight,' says the orthopod who's doing the job, 'lucky we didn't have to re-set it.' Not luck, just good management. For the first three or four minutes the nerves around the area of the break go into a trance. They become numb. That's when my builder mate and I managed to get it straight.

'Come back in three days for a check X-ray. If all's well it'll be off in three weeks.' Having wasted four and a half hours waiting to have it re-X-rayed on Tuesday, I lay on the table at work when the three weeks were up, and after a panel of four vets had viewed the rays we decided unanimously that the plaster be removed. I used to keep a picture on the X-ray viewer in the clinic. It was an interesting shot, taken by the hospital. The arm was in a sling at the time, and right where the fracture traversed the bone was the image of a dirty great safety pin. It, of course, simply held the sling in place, but you'd be surprised just how many clients asked why they used a safety pin to hold the two broken pieces of bone together.

It would be some ten years later that I'd become divorced from my first wife and by that time my young builder friend and his parents had moved north to that quiet little spot on the Clarence called Iluka. The whole separation and custody bit hit me pretty hard, and without the support of Janine through the whole thing I seriously doubt that my life would have panned out the way it has. Until you personally experience such a thing you will never understand the emotions and the sheer trauma of the undoing of so many years spent together. Friends and relatives are all so free with their advice on how to handle every situation. They should ask themselves just one question, 'Have I ever been through it?' If the answer is 'No', then keep your opinions to yourselves! As time goes by much of the bitterness ebbs away, and the memories that linger are, in the main, good ones. Time has a way of healing most wounds, but even with the best pair of surgical hands the years can employ there will always remain some sort of scar. Sometimes deep, usually shallow, but a scar nevertheless. It was Janine who encouraged a rather disconsolate vet to take his two children on their first holiday, a fishing trip, with only their father for company.

Iluka was the planned destination. My builder mate had erected a block of flats close to the water and his parents had moved in to manage the operation. We booked one for a fortnight. Tiffany was about ten and Russell some two years younger. The trip north took most of the day. Being only a dad you hope that the clothes and belongings you've packed are sufficient for the kids. As I struggled to lift the faithful old boat onto the roof of the station wagon with the supposed 'easy loader', I was beginning to wonder just how I'd manage everything when we got to the other end. Was I depressed? The answer is yes. Very much so. We even made a stop at Coffs Harbour and I bought a whole side of lamb, that way we would at least have something to eat. So sure was I that the whole experiment must go wrong!

It was after dark when we arrived. Everyone was tired and in need of a good night's sleep. The kids were fantastic. I believe they sensed what a trauma it was for me and pitched in to help like they'd never done before.

Next morning it was full-on. 'When can we go fishing?' they asked in unison, jumping wildly up and down with excitement. No point in postponing things, now was as good a time as any, and the tide looked about right. The Clarence is a big river and near its mouth on an outgoing run the water flows pretty quickly. Once or twice we'd fished the Iluka low wall, my wife and I. The water here was slower and quieter, and I mused that even if one of them did fall in they wouldn't get carried too far and hero Dad could yank them out. With lots of yells and screams from the kids and numerous scratches to the wagon's duco we managed to get the boat off the roof racks and into the water. The good old Mercury outboard was screwed onto the stern, fuel tank, rods, reels and bait loaded on board; now it was on with the life vests and the gumboots to prevent cuts from the oysters that grew in abundance on every rock of that wall.

In all honesty we could have rowed out. The water on the shore side was dead calm, and it was only a hundred metres or so out to the wall anyway. Carefully tying both bow and stern to the wall for extra stability, the kids soon scrambled ashore, both dead keen to catch their first fish. They were a lot more confident than their instructor.

'OK,' I explained slowly and carefully to my two students, 'fishing for blackfish is very different to fishing with a handline. These fish don't eat things like prawns, they eat weed,' I continued as the first rod and line began to take shape. 'Dad will bait it up and throw it out for you. Just watch the float as it moves slowly along in the water and when it goes under the water, that means a fish is eating your bait. Be sure to count . . . one . . . two . . . three, and then give your rod a sharp tug upwards and you'll hook him.' Sounds easy, doesn't it, but after years of practice and many hundreds of fish it still requires genuine skill.

In went the first cast of the day and I turned to rig up Tiffany's rod. About three-quarters of the way through the procedure I hear a very loud and confident 'one . . . two . . . three . . .' from Russell. Then a swish that becomes an audible 'thwack!' – that wonderful sound that only a greased floating line can make as it snaps taut between rod tip and float.

'I've got one. I've got one, Dad!'

Turning dismally around I could see the rod bent almost in half and a small child trying for all his worth to wind the reel. Here we go, I thought, every second cast they'll snag on something. Still you live in hope and feign encouragement.

'Well, just keep your rod tip up and wind him in,' I casually advised.

'Dad, I can't move it.'

Now I was absolutely certain that what he'd hooked was not a fish at all, but some dirty great lump of rock, sitting on the bottom, some five metres or so out in front of him. What a day this was going to be, nothing but tangled lines and re-rigging, I thought to myself.

'Dad, you've got to help me. I can't hold it!' By now his efforts to hold the rod anywhere near upright were fading, and quickly glancing around again for a second I thought the float surfaced and then dived vertically.

'Get the rod up. Get the tip up. Good boy.' Bloody hell, he had a fish on and a big one.

'I can't hold it, Dad. I can't!' It took just five seconds to get to his side. Standing behind your son while he hauls in his first luderick is something really special. A helping hand on the rod. Another helping hand to wind that beautiful Avon reel. Excitement levels are at a maximum. The float is going wild, dancing and diving in a frantic ballet as the fish not yet visible fights against the tiny hook in its upper jaw. Time is forgotten, the contest is sensational. The rod is working overtime, its tip flexing and bending, lending its support to the competition. The landing net slides under our first fish of the day. It's well over a kilo, wet, slippery and bronze, glistening in the morning sunshine. There are celebrations all round. Everyone is dancing and I'm doing a quickstep. Sen-bloody-sational!

He caught another four, his sister three, that's a total of eight. 'That'll do us, won't it, Dad? That's plenty for tea, isn't it?' How can you argue with the logic of children? I didn't even get my line in the water! That afternoon the flat owners returned after a weekend away. They were enthused by the news of our success. Next day it was an all-out effort. Three adults and two kids equalled forty-four fish; thankfully, a few were mine. The day after, their son and a mate joined us. The kids elected to stay home and watch a bit of telly with the lady of the house. The four of us got eighty! That was it. We tried again on other days, but they just weren't there. That's the way it goes with fishing. Here today and gone tomorrow.

What a top holiday it proved to be. Every night we ate fish pieces cooked in egg and breadcrumbs with the Cooper family's famous saratoga chips on the side. In fact, we never ate one morsel of that side of lamb. As far as I know my landlords consumed that lot after we left. Funnily enough, a holiday that I began with such a feeling of impending doom turned out to be one of the most memorable of all. Thanks, darling!

34

Rawhide Rick

Back in the days of Mole Creek, the farm and all those sheep, our daughter Heidi at the age of about five attended the local convent school in Deloraine. It truly was a beautiful little school and we've been back there since to do a story for 'Harry's Practice', about a galah, with one of the classes.

As a parent there's always that feeling of concern when your child arrives home with a note asking you to ring the teacher. Such was the occasion this particular Tuesday. Janine and I mulled over the letter wondering what on earth was the matter. It was no good asking Heidi, she was totally oblivious to the whole affair.

'Anything special happen at school today, darling?' Janine asked.

'No, Mummy, nothing special, we just talked about what happened on our holidays.'

'Sure there was nothing else?' asked Janine again.

A shake of the head was the only reply.

It was my habit to drop our daughter at school on the way to work at my veterinary clinic and her teacher was always there a good thirty minutes prior to the start of the school day.

'Could I see you for a minute?' I asked Mary Owens. 'It's about the note you sent home'.

'Sure, but you'd better come into the office so we can have some privacy.' The note was now taking on a somewhat serious aspect. 'Could you tell me a little about what you did in Sydney over the holiday weekend?'

'Sure,' I said. Going back to Sydney where we had literally been born and bred was a very different experience once we'd spent even a couple of years away from the place. It was like being a tourist. Shopping. Exploring, riding a train, a trip to Manly on the ferry. Even a trip around town on the Monorail.

'Oh yes,' she said, 'what happened on the Monorail?'

'Well,' I said, 'we never got to ride the darn thing when we lived there, so we bought a ticket and the three of us simply travelled around getting off at every station. Most of them are pretty boring, but one place Heidi loved.'

I went on to describe a station down at the bottom end of town. There were very few shops, but there was a bar, an eatery, and a large amusement parlour right inside. We had a soft drink and Heidi was in seventh heaven with all the machines, the bright lights, the silver balls, the flashing, the numbers; you name it, nothing like this at Mole Creek. Drinks over and having played a game or two of pinball, we were walking out when one particular device caught Heidi's attention.

'Look at that, Dad, look at that!' She was pointing at a large screen with a rather disreputable looking cowboy, arms folded, staring meanly down with cold steely eyes set in an unshaven and menacing face.

'Betchya can't out-gun me.' The image challenged all and sundry.

'Go on, Dad, you could beat him, betchya could.'

Sometimes the challenge, or is it the temptation, to be a kid again is just too great. Sod it, I'll give it a go. We were on holidays, let's have a good time. (The times weren't too good on the farm.)

The set-up was something like this. You stood with a gun

on a stand approximating your left or your right hip. It was electronically controlled with a cord attached. There were three degrees of difficulty, I chose the mid-range. Money in the slot, pressed the go button and the cowboy on the screen starts to look even more menacing.

'You reckon you can outdraw ol' Rawhide Rick? No one outdraws ol' Rawhide Rick, and not some greenhorn like you, I'm a gonna count to three, when we get to three, if you can count that far you draw and fire, 'cause I'll be drawin' too!' Heidi was right beside me riveted to the screen, watching every move this electronic gunslinger made, a few more insulting remarks and then the countdown.

'One . . . two . . . three!'

My right hand closed over the handle of the revolver. It slid quickly and easily from the holster, was up into position and fired with all the speed I could muster.

'A lucky shot . . . a lucky shot, that's all, I'll be back, you've got one more go . . . only one of us leaves this place alive.'

Heidi gripped my left arm like a vice. 'Don't miss him, Dad, only one of you is going to live!'

'Don't worry, darling.' I was now as much a part of the action as the damned game could possibly entice.

'You were lucky last time, this time it's my turn, this time I'll be faster, you'd better be faster too!'

'You can be faster, can't you, Daddy?'

'I'll try, darling, I'll try.' The ol' heart's really pumping, even the right hand feels a bit sweaty.

'Don't touch that gun yet!' My hand simply brushed over the handle.

'I ain't started countin' yet.' I'm even opening and closing my hand in anticipation. This is ridiculous.

'One . . . two . . . three!'

Somehow the revolver cleared the holster even more easily than before and as the barrel came up into line with his chest, the trigger finger reached maximum tension . . . bang!!!

'You got him, Dad . . . You got him . . . You beauty!!!'

'You got me, you mongrel, you're too good for me, I'm goin' to Boot Hill now, I'm gone, but one day one of my kin will be back and he'll be lookin' for you.' The screen goes blank, a green hill and a cross appear with the simple inscription – 'out-gunned, but not out-done'.

Kids believe whatever they want to believe. You can tell your children many things, but in spite of all we may or may not do, they form their own opinions based on events that occur around them. In other words, it's not what you say as a parent, but rather what you do. Heidi had put her very own interpretation upon the events of that afternoon; it, in fact, had been the highlight of her whole trip to Sydney.

Tuesday was news day for her class and what was Heidi's news? I'll quote it verbatim: 'Mrs Owens, Daddy shot a man in a bar.'

35

Cooper's Mob

After Mole Creek and a period of time renting, we'd scraped together enough cash and told enough lies to get into a house of our own again at Relbia. We hadn't been in the place five minutes when the boss decided we needed a change of livestock. Although the property was set up mainly to handle our Welsh and Australian ponies we had managed to hang on to a few of the pet sheep we had hand-raised back in that first horrible lambing season at The Den. The treasure of all these, and still going today, was Mary, a somewhat squat Suffolk Polwarth cross.

'I've always liked British alpine goats,' began Janine's dinnertime conversation. Yeah, I knew that. Her pet goat had been mauled by a dog and I'd put the poor thing down for her, way back in the Annangrove days, before we actually met. This conversation was the softening-up process that always preceded the purchase of some new animal.

'I've ordered a pair of them, they'll be here in the morning.'

'What do we need goats for?' I asked, rather incredulously.

'I just like them.' You cannot argue with that sort of logic.

First there were two, a nanny and a neutered male, then another just mysteriously appeared, and another rogue female some two months later that no one could get near even with a bucket of feed! The first two had been hand-raised and were great pets. They would follow you round the place like dogs. But there is one major problem with goats. They have no regard at all for fences, unless they are electric. Ours were not. They are great browsers and some experts suggest that goats with their habit of eating everything are responsible for the great deserts of the world. They certainly set about turning our paddocks into a similar landscape – then not content with that, simply jumped the fences into next door and continued on their path of destruction. Our then neighbour had stud Charolais cattle, and a stray goat or two meant nothing to him. Finally after all this fence-vaulting, the boundary collapsed and the sheep joined in the fray. It was an embarrassment to find half your stock merrily munching their way through the next-door neighbour's river flats!

Things would be different at 'Arcadian Downs' – but they weren't. The fences were in better shape but still nowhere near good enough for a goat determined to get to somewhere it shouldn't be. Our neighbour was a tolerant man. 'Mate, those damn goats are in my oat paddock again,' this was the third phone call in as many weeks, and all credit to her, it was Janine who said, 'They'll have to go.'

The question always is, of course, where do they go?

'I reckon we should just put them through Killafaddy saleyards.'

'Yes, but how will I know who buys them?'

'Does it really matter?' I exclaimed, fairly frustrated.

'Yes, it does matter. And when you take them, take those rotten wethers of yours as well.' This was developing into a bit of a tit for tat, but not wanting to rock the boat, I agreed. The mob of sheep had now expanded to something like seventeen. Mary and Inky were the two pets. Then there was a group of multicoloured ewes that Janine had bought from our good friend Geoff just because she liked them, and some of their offspring, four of whom were as mad as rabid snakes. You could not do one thing with them.

Tuesday was sale day. I had rung and booked our lot with the local agent, who was probably still laughing the next morning after Janine had lectured him on getting the details of our goat buyers so she could follow up to see how they'd settled in. The goats were easy to catch, by now even the nutcase would come when the boss called. One at a time they were led up into the back of the horse float. That's the easy part, I thought, now for the sheep. Once again the whole place was set up for horses, not sheep. It's a totally different fencing system, which the sheep adapted to very quickly. They would simply duck under the lowest electric wire and with all that wool they were completely insulated. Anything else would have got zapped! Rosie was still on the go, and with her help and the portable sheep panels we'd held on to after Mole Creek, we eventually got the mob into the horse yards. These are solid wooden structures that would probably hold a bull elephant, so they certainly held the sheep.

'I'll sort out the four that are going, and run them up into the race, if you can man the gate.' Janine shook her head in acknowledgment, and stood by the big gate that separated the main yard from the smaller holding yard in which we now had the mob. One at a time I eased the sheep we were keeping through the gate. Things were going well. There were only two left to separate. The gate was open no more than two feet. I stood squarely in the middle, and this darn ugly maniac of a Suffolk cross wether in full wool was staring me down. Most sheep will back off. Not this one. He could see his mates on the other side and that's where he wanted to be as well. Only yours truly stood in the way. He stamped the front foot. Lowered the head in a mock charge and then charge he did. Right into my left shin. Head down, he caught me right smack in the middle of bone.

'Bloody hell!' and I half-sank to the ground, while he went back for another go at me. Janine swung the gate shut.

'Are you all right?'

'No. I think the bastard's broken me bloody leg.' The pain was unbelievable. 'I'll be OK. Just give me a hand to put this lot into the race and I'll get them one at a time and chuck them in the front of the float.' Somehow we managed to get all four sheep into the horse race. It's fairly narrow, horses can't turn around in it, but the bloody sheep could. I hobbled in, with Rosie behind, caught the first one by a hind leg, rolled him over on the side and began to drag the wretched animal out into the open. To cope with horses, the race and all the yard fences were two metres high and at each end of the race was a metal gate, constructed from fifty millimetre square tube. Built for a purpose, it had horizontal bars spaced every 450 millimetres. Janine stood by the gate ready to close it just as soon as I had wrestled the first wether through. It was, if I remember, only about one-third open, Janine could shut it quickly if needs be. The wether had other ideas. Just as the struggling animal all but cleared the race he flipped over onto his back, his rump slammed into the gate and sent it flying violently backward right to where my poor wife was standing. The horizontal steel tube collected her squarely above her right eye with a sickening thud and she fell to the ground in a heap.

Holding onto the cursed animal with one hand, shutting the gate with the other and yelling for help from Linda, our kennel girl, I just had to leave Janine in her care for a moment until the protesting ovine was ensconced safely in the front of the float. Hobbling back on one leg, I revived Janine and assisted my poor wife from the scene of battle. Ice was produced and colour gradually returned to her face, as the size of the egg above her eye grew bigger. It was even Stevens as to who was in the most pain, but sometimes pain drives you on and there was no way these four damn sheep were going to beat me. Between us, Rosie and I somehow managed to skull-drag the other three victims across the open yard and into the horse float.

'Will you be OK if I go?'

'Yes, just damn well go and get them out of here!'

It's a twenty-minute drive to the saleyards and all the way there I'm sure the leg is broken. There's a spot for trailers and the like so I pull up there. The agent comes over to say g'day. I open the door, step out of the car and fall flat on my face. Suddenly the leg just won't take any weight at all. Help arrives. In ten minutes it's all over: the wethers are yarded, the goats march off happily on their leads and I crawl back into the car for the trip home. Janine is up at the house with a huge ice pack on her forehead, lying buried in cushions on the lounge. I can use only one leg, the other is already swollen to nearly half again its normal size. More ice! We both took the day off.

The corollary is even more interesting. Next Monday it's the last Rotary meeting before Christmas. There's my darling wife all dolled up, but with one magnificent shiner obliterating her eye completely. Yours truly is still on only one leg (never did get it X-rayed, but I'm sure I cracked it) – all and sundry thought we'd had a major domestic! Then Christmas Day itself; both of us still looking like we'd gone a round or two with

Muhammad Ali. It took five weeks for her eye to recover and three months for my leg to come good. We got $22 each for the goats and, yes, they all went to the one home. The wethers brought $13.20 each and that's probably $13 more than any of them were worth.

We still have a dozen sheep and every year it's the joke of the neighbourhood. It takes seven men and four dogs to bring Cooper's mob in to be shorn. Nothing ever changes. Really. Does it?

36

Polly and the Nursing Homes

Polly the possum was rescued by our friends Rudy and Barb after her mother was flattened on the road just outside where they used to live in Ulverstone. She had a badly damaged left front foot, and even now has trouble gripping, so would not survive in the wild. By our calculations she's at least twelve years old and still Janine is the only one who can comfortably handle her. I've got the scars to prove that!

She was a beaut to rear, sucked the formula from the word go. Her funniest trick was to greet me at the door when I got back from the surgery. I'd take two steps inside with a pair of moleskins on, and this little marsupial must have reckoned I looked like some sort of gum tree. She would race across the floor and spring at my leg, landing somewhere just above the knee and in a flash would be sitting on my head. With time, this became a rather painful experience.

'Let's cut her claws,' I suggested, displaying the scratches all over my upper torso. Janine agreed, and we trimmed front and back; they were really sharp. Next night, I arrive home from work, same routine. Polly flies across the floor, makes the usual leap, lands and proceeds to slide vertically down my leg.

'Look what you've done to her,' screams Janine, 'she can't climb any more!'

It only took three days for things to return to normal.

Once we got settled in Relbia, Janine decided that it might

be something of a community service if she were to visit one or two of the nursing homes around the area. All concerned thought this a great idea and with the help of a girlfriend or, on occasions, Heidi, she would head off with a car full of just about everything on the property except a horse. There were rabbits, guinea pigs, rats, fantail pigeons, kittens, cats, dogs and of course the odd wombat and Polly the poss. It was quite an expedition. Even Pol was well trained, Janine could take her out on the back lawn, tickle her in just the right spot and she'd go, as everyone should do before they travel. Let's face it, possum urine stinks!

On arrival Janine would be greeted by the staff and helped in with all the cages before she began her usual talk. Visits lasted upwards of an hour, and my darling wife would take great pains to explain the feeding and behaviour patterns of all the animals she had on display. In the main all the cast were well behaved, with the odd exception of Polly. Janine would carry her on her shoulder, the possum's furry tail wrapped around her right hand for control. But you daren't walk under any low-slung plant material, Polly would make an instant leap and land in whatever hanging basket seemed to be nearby, whether real or artificial. (This possum gets better fed than you and me. Cereal, sweetcorn, tomatoes, carrots, celery, raw almonds, broccoli, strawberries, kiwifruit – and in season, blueberries, her absolute favourite! It's extremely dangerous to walk anywhere near Polly if you're wearing earrings that in any way resemble, in either colour or shape, the aforementioned morsel. Many a poor lady has had them ripped from her earlobes by an over-inquisitive possum, and, boy, is she quick.)

Many of these homes present some really sad cases, and the

occupational therapist often asks Janine to spend just a little extra time at the end of her talk with one or two individuals. This is her favourite story, and mine too!

'He had a stroke about nine months ago and ever since then he's just sat in his wheelchair and no one seems to be able to get through to him at all,' advised the matron. 'Do you think you could try, Janine?'

Of course she'd try. Heidi was with her, helping to gather up all the animals. You had to be careful to count all the kittens before you started, some of the little old ladies had a habit of secreting one or two under their knee rugs. Janine walked over. 'Hello, how are you?' There was no response. 'Would you like to nurse a kitten?' She put one on his lap.

'What about a rat?' And she let Felix, her favourite, run up the arm of his pyjamas. Not a movement. Much the same with everything she tried, she even let Polly slither up his legs and onto his shoulder. Still the old man sat there head down, speechless as if his body no longer encased any real spark of life. She'd all but given up, all the animals were back in their cages, dogs on their leads, and on their way out to the car. All that remained were two fantail pigeons still strutting their stuff proudly round and round in the centre of the floor. Pigeons are birds with plenty of brains, but I fear that fantails lost some of theirs the moment they started throwing their heads back.

As if it were a casual gesture she threw one of the birds in the direction of this man. It hovered for just a second above him and then fluttered down as fantails do and landed squarely on his lap, immediately throwing itself into the usual head-back, fan-out position. Janine turned to retrieve the bird, but stopped instantly. Something fantastic was happening. She's said to me time and time again, 'It's as though someone turned on the lights.' It took nearly twenty minutes for two feeble, almost greying, hands that had not moved for nine months to find their way onto his lap. Another ten to grasp the bird. He held the bird like a true pigeon fancier, the way we've all been taught, with both legs gripped firmly between the first and second finger of the right hand and the bird's breast cradled in the palm. His grip was weak, but the bird seemed to know, it sat there as the other hand stroked the wings and fanned the tail. Tears ran down his cheeks and fell in pools on the bird. The man's colour had changed from a sombre grey to a pink and healthy tone. He struggled to lift his head. Janine looked up from where she knelt on the floor, held his hands in hers and saw a smile crease his face.

As a young man in Europe he had raced pigeons. He knew what they were. He knew instinctively how to handle a bird. Just a bird, one of God's small feathered creatures, had unlocked the door and let the light shine again. If this was to be the only success that Janine's many visits were ever to have, then every one of them has been worthwhile. One little bird, a small black and white fantailed pigeon . . . one little bird made all the difference.

As a vet I feel proud that today right throughout the medical and nursing professions there has been at last a recognition of the fantastic role that animals can play in helping the human population cope with mental and physical health-related disabilities. Janine and I will continue to do our bit to help promote the work done by such organisations as the guide dogs, assistance dogs, pets as therapy animals, and the thousands of volunteers who so regularly visit hospitals, nursing homes and hospices to bring laughter and companionship to people in need.

A life without an animal would be a very empty one. Our life is full to the brim!

Dr Harry Cooper
Anecdotes & Antidotes

Dr Harry Cooper, Australia's favourite vet and much-loved star of 'Harry's Practice', has a lifetime's worth of stories to tell about his experiences with animals and their owners.

From hilarious accounts of dysfunctional birds and cunning canines, to moving tales of the loss of childhood pets, *Anecdotes & Antidotes* is a collection of these very special stories, told with Dr Harry's trademark warmth and humour.

In the tradition of *All Creatures Great and Small*, *Anecdotes & Antidotes* will enthral not only animal lovers, but anyone who enjoys a good yarn.